SEM PICTORIAL GUIDE TO TREMATODES OF LIVESTOCK AND POULTRY IN INDIA

Veena Tandon
and
Bishnupada Roy
Department of Zoology,
North-Eastern Hill University,
Shillong 793 022, India

Regency Publications
NEW DELHI

FRONT COVER: *Paramphistomum epiclitum*, anterior region of body.

ISBN 81-87498-59-5

Published by Regency Publications, 20/36-G, Old Market, West Patel Nagar, New Delhi 110 008 for North-Eastern Hill University, Shillong, and Printed at Radiant Printers, New Delhi 110 008, Phones: 571 2539. 574 0038; Telefax: 578 3571.

Email: regency@satyam.net.in

Preface

An exhaustive survey of helminth parasites in the livestock, i.e., cattle, buffalo, sheep, goat, pig and poultry, in some of the north eastern states of India by the authors revealed a wide spectrum of trematode species occurring in them. In view of the apparent morphological similarity among many of these parasite species, it seemed that fine morphological features may exhibit species-specific patterns and thus may be of diagnostic value. The present collection of pictures illustrates surface fine topographical features as revealed through the scanning electron microscopy and is an outcome of the attempt to provide an authentic inventory of the components of the spectrum of digenean parasites occurring in the mentioned host animals of the region.

We are grateful to the Editors of the journals *Zoologischer Anzeiger, Revista di Parasitologia, Acta Parasitologica Polonica, Journal of Helminthology, Parasitology Research, Indian Journal of Parasitology (now Journal of Parasitic Diseases)*, for their permission to reproduce some of the electron micrographs published earlier in their respective journals. Our thanks are due to the Head, Department of Zoology, North-Eastern Hill University, Shillong for providing necessary laboratory facilities and to Regional Sophisticated Instrumentation Centre, under the auspices of NEHU, for the use of the SEM facility. We are indebted to Mr. Bijoy Das for printing the photographs. The research grant of the project, 'Screening to Edible Host Animals in the North-Eastern Region for Helminth Parasitic Infections and Their Plausible Role in Zoonoses in Human Population'—sponsored by the North-East Council Government of India, to one of us (VT), provided the much needed financial support for the field collections of the parasites, which is thankfully acknowledged. We also acknowledge the help of Bioinformatics Centre (sponsored by Department of Biotechnology, Ministry of Science & Technology, GOI) at NEHU and support from 'All India Coordinated Project on Capacity Building in Taxonomy: Research on Helminths' (sponsored to VT by Ministry of Environment & Forests, GOI) towards the completion of this work.

It is our hope that this pictorial guide would serve as an easy tool for students, teachers, researchers and all those working with the trematode parasites of the economically important livestock.

Veena Tandon
Bishnupada Roy

Preface

Contents

Contents

Introduction

Digenetic trematodes constitute an important group of helminth parasites which pose a continual and unacceptable threat to the life of their hosts. Animals like sheep, goats, cattle, buffaloes, pigs and poultry form a considerable source of food for human population. While parasites infecting these animals make them unfit for human consumption, at the same time they also cause a steady drain on their vitality and growth resulting in their high rate of mortality leading to immense losses to animal-based economic ventures.

For the last three decades a lot of work has been done pertaining to the spectrum and prevalence of digenetic trematodes in livestock animals in different parts of India. In his treatise on digenetic trematodes of vertebrates, Yamaguti (1971) listed 41 families of Digenea occurring in mammals. Of these, those parasitizing the livestock like cattle, buffalo, sheep, goat and pig in different parts of the globe represent 10 families. Yamaguti recognised 25 genera as represented in the Indian livestock. These genera are: *Schistosoma* Weinland, 1858; *Orientobilharzia* Dutt et Srivastava, 1955; *Paramphistomum* Fischoeder, 1901; *Calicophoron* Näsmark, 1937; *Cotylophoron* Stiles et Goldberger, 1910; *Olveria* Thapar et Sinha, 1945; *Homalogaster* Poirier, 1883; *Gastrodiscus* Leuckart, 1877; *Gastrodiscoides* Leiper, 1913; *Orthocoelium* (Stiles et Goldberger, 1910) Price et McIntosh, 1953; *Gastrothylax* Poirier, 1883; *Carmyerius* Stiles et Goldberger, 1910; *Fischoederius* Stiles et Goldberger, 1910; *Johnsonitrema*, Yamaguti, 1958; *Ogmocotyle* Skrjabin et Schultz, 1933; *Fasciola* Linnaeus, 1758; *Fasciolopsis* Looss, 1899; *Echinostoma* Rudolphi, 1809; *Artyfechinostomum* Lane, 1915; *Dicrocoelium* Dujardin, 1845; *Eurytrema* Looss, 1907; *Paragonimus* Braun, 1899; *Opisthorchis* Blanchard, 1895; *Amphimerus* Barker, 1911 and *Clonorchis* Looss, 1907. Of these genera, while most are common to other parts of the world, the genus *Olveria* is totally endemic to India and *Artyfechinostomum* is also confined to the Indian sub-continent, though also reported from neighbouring Malayan region (Mehra, 1980). *Echinostoma* and *Catatropis* Odhner, 1905 are the common digenetic genera represented in the poultry.

In the last two decades, several new genera and species of digenetic trematodes from Indian ruminant and swine hosts have been described; also some new records of species were added. Singh (1970) described *Cochinocotyle bovini*, a new genus and new species, from rumen of cattle. Bambroo (1970) described a new species of *Gastrothylax* from sheep in Kashmir. Varghese et al. (1971) reported the occurrence of the heterophyid, *Haplorchis taichui* (Nishigori, 1924) in domestic pigs. Bali and Fotedar (1974) recorded and described a new species of *Olveria* from the rumen of sheep in Kashmir. Srivastava et al. (1980) added a new genus and new species, *Duttiella cephaloporus*, to the list of amphistomids of the Indian ruminants. However, the validity of many of these taxa has been questioned by subsequent authors (ref. revisions of the paramphistomid families and other taxa by Sey, 1979–1985; Eduardo, 1980–1985; Jones, 1986; Mehra, 1980 and Srivastava, 1982). Three more new species, namely *Velasquezotrema tripurensis*, *Leiperocotyle meghalayensis* and *Calicophoron shillongensis* were described from ruminant hosts by Roy and Tandon (1990a, b; 1995). Many of these species, amphistomes in particular, appear morphologically similar on gross visual and light microscopic examination. Identification of these species, when based on histological criteria, becomes a tedious task. In this context, scanning electron microscopy has now emerged as an important reliable tool in the morphological and taxonomic studies. The present pictorial guide is a presentation of scanning electron micrographs depicting surface morphological features of digenetic trematodes commonly parasitizing the livestock and poultry in Northeast India. The taxonomic classification of the genera and species given herein mainly follows Eduardo (1980–1985) and Srivastava (1982). In respect of amphistomid parasites, generalised organisation of the pharynx, genital atrium and acetabulum has been included, with a definition of the various organisational types of these structures, so as to provide the supplementary diagnostic characters which are at present being used conventionally.

The materials used for the SEM studies were all freshly collected from the abattoirs of the various places in the region. The specimens were fixed in 10% neutral buffered formalin (NBF) or 2.5% Glutaraldehyde followed by post fixation in 1% Osmium tetraoxide, dehydrated through ascending series of acetone or alcohol and dried in a critical-point-drier using liquid carbon dioxide as the drying medium. In lieu of the critical-point drying, the specimens were also treated with Tetramethylsilane (TMS), following Dey et al. (1989). The dried specimens were fixed on to the stubs using colloidal silver or double-sided adhesive tape, metal-coated with gold palladium and observed under a Jeol 35 CF Scanning electron microscope.

Genus : *Schistosoma* Winland, 1858
Host : *Bos indicus*, *Bubalus bubalis*
Habitat : Blood vessels
Species : *Schistosoma indicum* Montgomery, 1906

(Figs. 1–5 male; 6–8 female)

Specific characters:

Intestine bifurcating at level of ventral sucker, reuniting in posterior one-third region of body and continuing as single caecum for shot distance. In male, testes clustered, 6–12 in number, close behind ventral sucker. In female, ovary behind level of mid-body, 21–27 eggs in uterus.

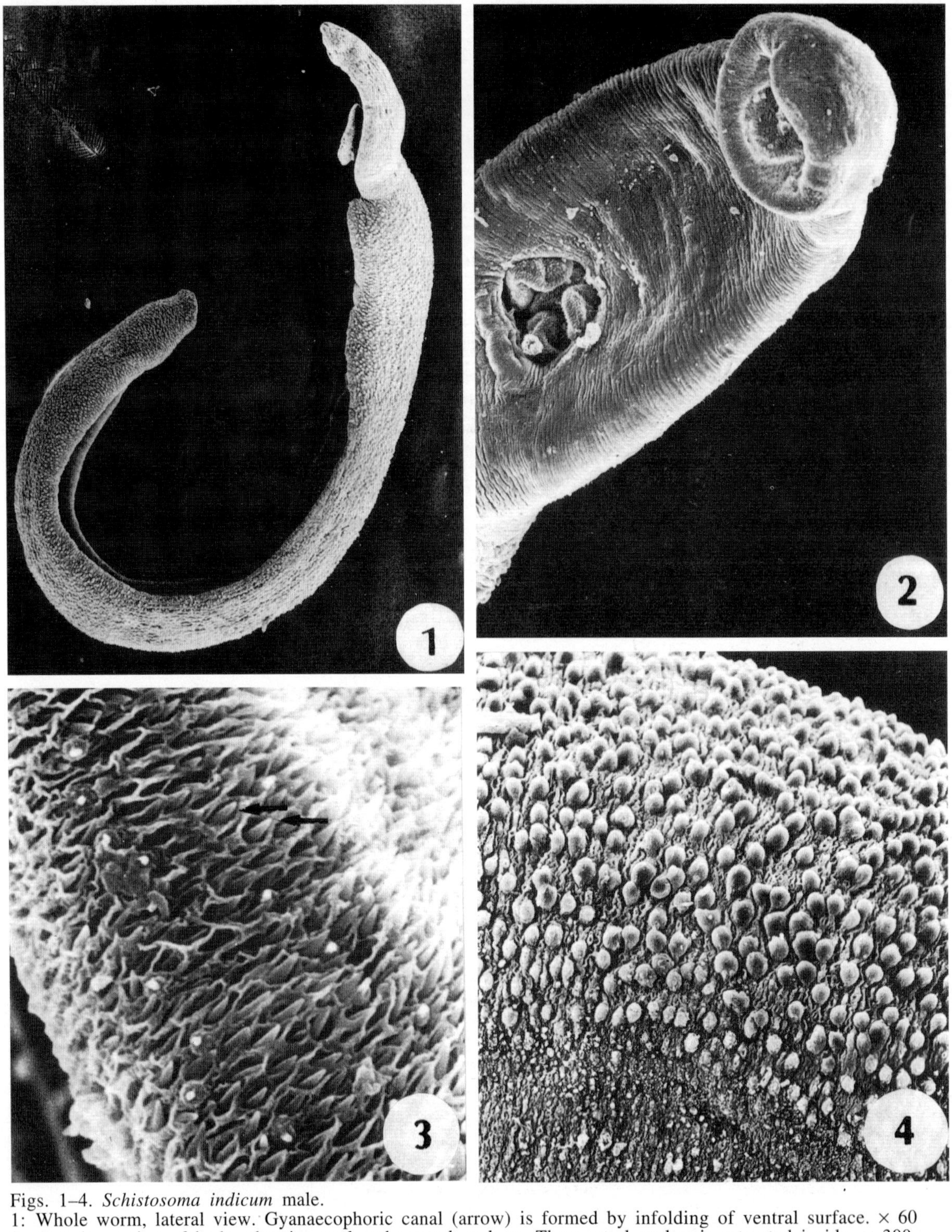

Figs. 1–4. *Schistosoma indicum* male.
1: Whole worm, lateral view. Gyanaecophoric canal (arrow) is formed by infolding of ventral surface. × 60
2: Anterior region of body, showing oral and ventral suckers. The ventral sucker is retracted inside. × 300
3: A part of oral sucker in an enlarged view. Note the spines, each lodged in a cavity (arrows). × 4000
4: Tegument of dorsal surface, showing clustered smooth and round papillae. × 540

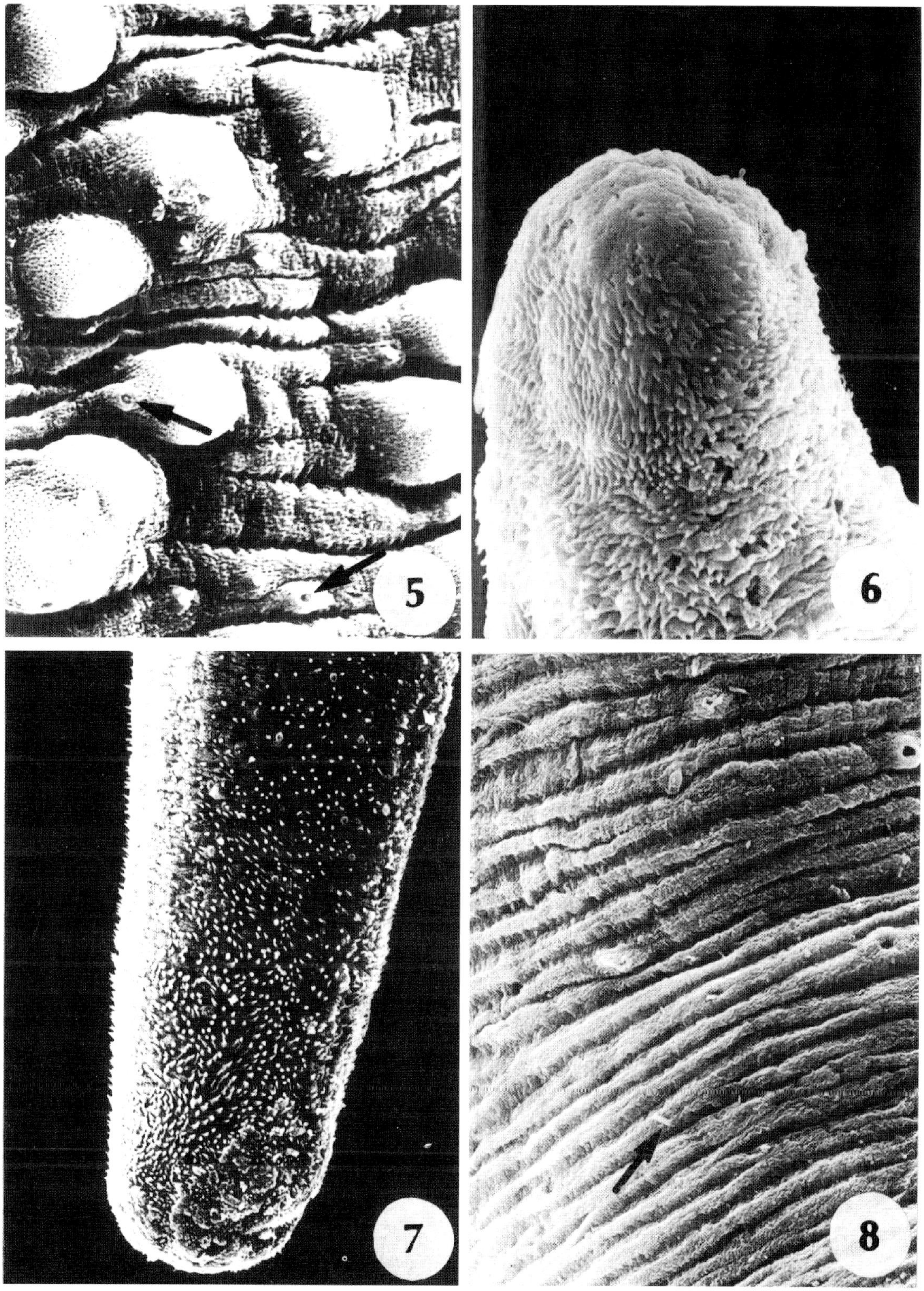

Figs. 5–8. *Schistosoma indicum.*

5: Male—enlarged view of dorsal surface, showing tegumental pitted papillae (arrows) and numerous minute punctations. × 2600

6: Anterior region of body of female worm with posteriorly directed spines, which help in anchorage with the male gynaecophoric canal. × 2000

7: Posterior region of body, showing densely packed spines. × 1000

8: A closer view of general body surface in middle region of body, showing sparsely distributed spines (arrows) and tegumental pits. × 2000

Genus : *Paramphistomum* Fischoeder, 1901
Host : *Bos indicus*, *Bubalus bubalis*, *Ovis aries*, *Capra hircus*
Species : *Paramphistomum epiclitum* Fischoeder, 1904
[Syn. *Paramphistomum indicum* Stiles et Goldberger, 1910 in part
Paramphistomum thapari Price et McIntosh, 1953
Cotylophoron indicum Stiles et Goldberger, 1910
Cotylophoron madrasense Gupta, 1958
Srivastavaia indica Singh, 1970]

(Figs. 9–12)

Specific characters:

Pharynx of calicophoron type (internal surface lined by small domed papillae), without anterior sphincter; vitellaria not confluent dorsomedially; testes deeply lobed; terminal genitalium of epiclitum type (having a wall which is semicircular in outline like a sucker); acetabulum of paramphistomum type (dorsoexternal circular muscles (d.e.c.m.) divided into two parts: d.e.c.m. 1 and d.e.c.m. 2), acetabular rim having no posterior notch.

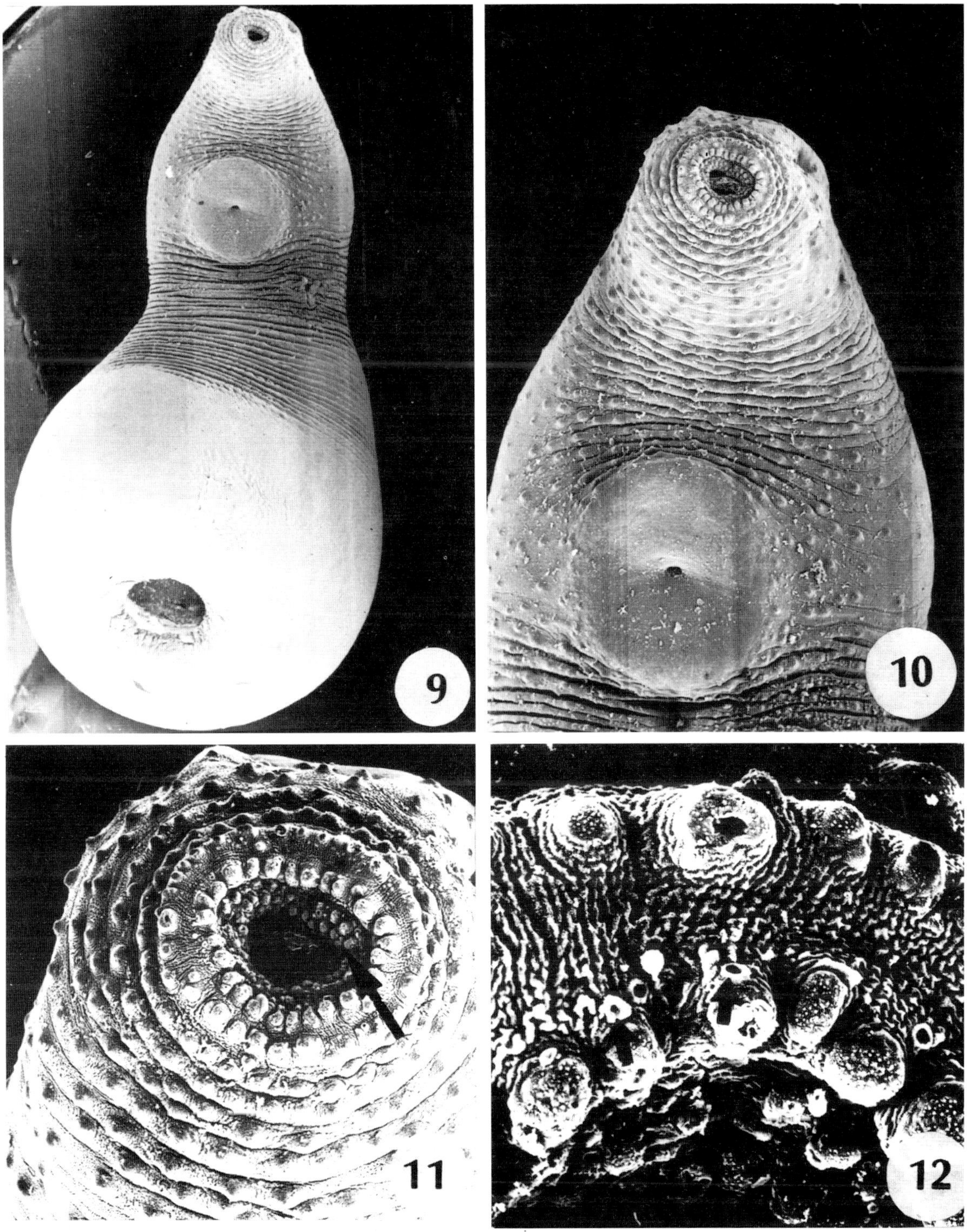

Figs. 9–12. *Paramphistomum epiclitum*.
9: Whole worm, ventral view. × 20
10: Anterior region of body, showing arrangement of papillae around the oral aperture and genital pore opening. × 44
11: Oral end enlarged, showing circles of papillae around the oral aperture and at the inner wall of pharynx (arrow). × 200
12: A closer view of circum-oral papillae. Both pitted and non-pitted ciliated papillae are present in two rows at the rim; numerous minute pits (arrows) are also present in between the two rows of papillae. × 540

Species : *Paramphistomum gracile* Fischoeder, 1901
[Syn. *Paramphistomum indicum* Stiles et Goldberger,1910, in part
Paramphistomum bombayiensis Gupta et Verma in Gupta et Nakhasi, 1977
Paramphistomum ichikawai of Gupta et Nakhasi (1977)]

(Figs. 13–16)

Specific Characters:

Pharynx of calicophoron type, having no anterior sphincter; vitellaria not confluent dorsomedially; testes deeply lobed; terminal genitalia of gracile type (with well developed genital papilla); acetabulum of paramphistomum type.

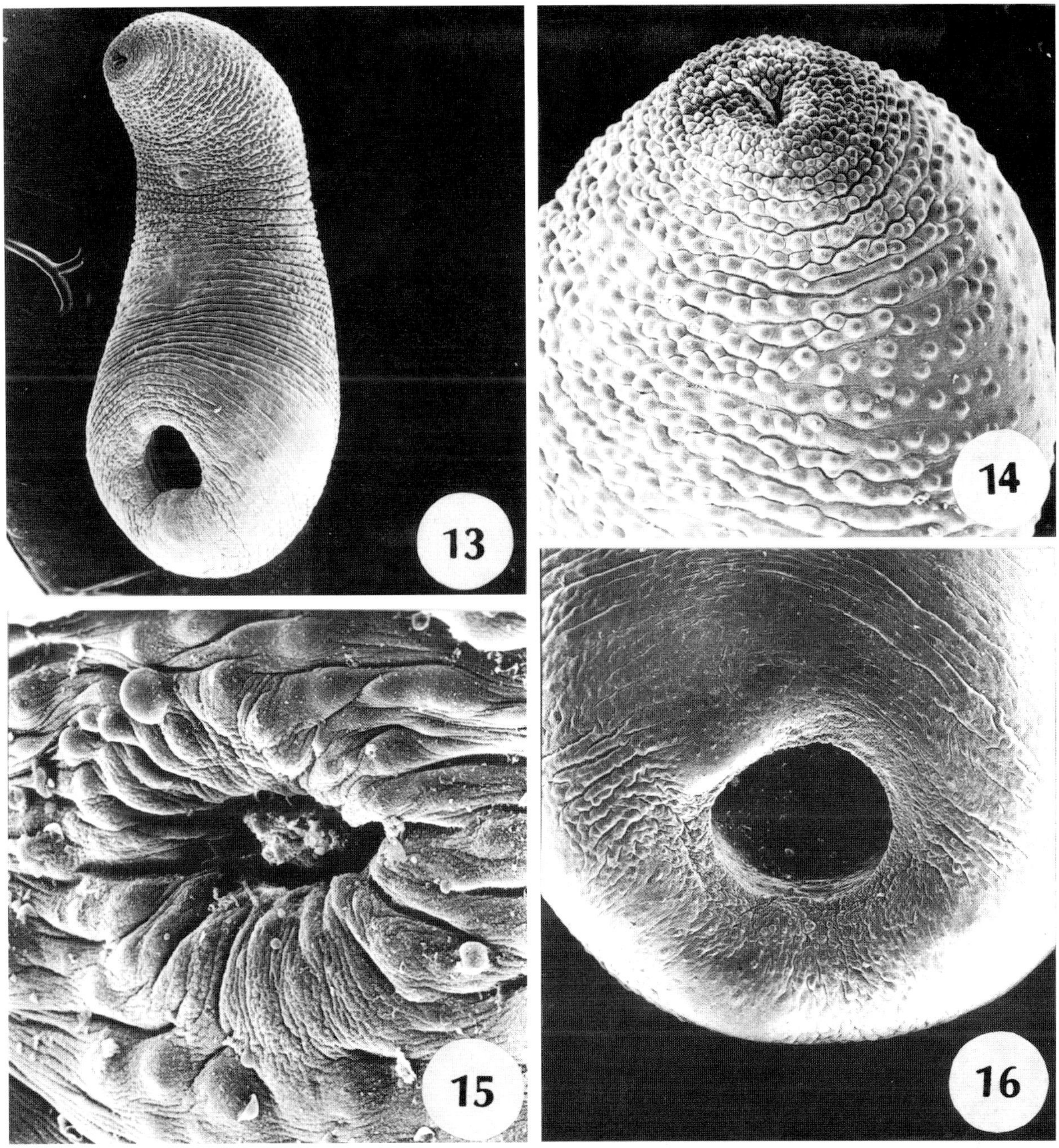

Figs. 13–16. *Paramphistomum gracile.*
13: Whole worm, ventral view. × 20
14: Anterior end, showing dense aggregation of smooth, domed papillae. × 78
15: Genital pore region indicating radial tegumental foldings and dome-like tuberculations. × 480
16: Acetabular region. × 48

Genus : *Calicophoron* Näsmark, 1932
Host : B*os indicus*, *Bubalus bubalis*, *Ovis aries*, *Capra hircus*
Habitat : Rumen
Species : *Calicophoron calicophorum* (Fischoeder, 1901) Näsmark, 1937
[Syn. *Paramphistomum calicophorum* Fischoeder, 1901
Paramphistomum crassum Stiles et Goldberger, 1910
Paramphistomum cauliorchis Stiles et Goldberger, 1910
Paramphistomum ijimai Fukui, 1922
Paramphistomum (*cauliorchis*) Skrjabini Popora, 1937
Paramphistomum erschovi Davydora, 1959
Calicophoron orientalis Mukherjee, 1966
Calicophoron skrjabini Mitskevich, 1958]

(Figs. 17–20)

Specific Characters:

True ventral atrium absent; pharynx of calicophoron type; terminal genitalium of calicophoron type (presence of genital pillar in everted condition, with genital pore opening at tip); acetabulum of calicophoron type (d.e.c.m. and ventral exterior circular muscles (v.e.c.m.) not divided into two parts, dorsal and ventral halves of exterior circular muscles (e.c.m.) practically identical).

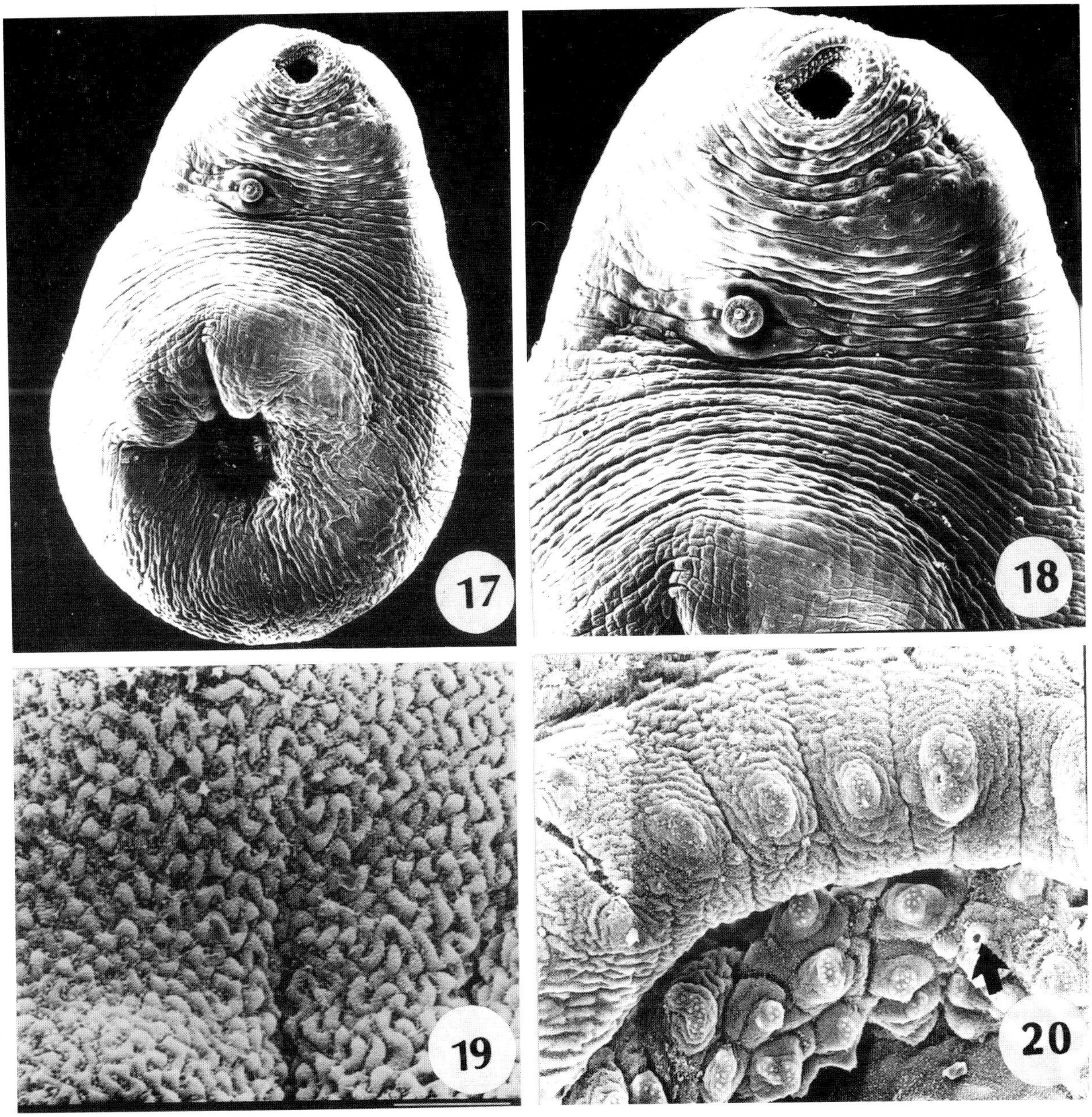

Figs. 17–20. *Calicophoron calicophorum*.
17: Whole worm, ventral view. × 26
18: Anterior end of body; note the circular ridges with domed papillae surrounding the oral aperture and protruded genital papilla. × 48
19: Surface tegument, enlarged view showing fine tegumental foldings. × 140
20: Rim of oral sucker and inner wall of buccal cavity, showing ciliated papillae at the rim and in the inner wall of pharynx; the inner wall is also provided with pits (arrow). × 660

Species : *Calicophoron papillosum* (Stiles et Goldberger, 1910) Näsmark, 1937
[Syn. *Paramphistomum papillosum* Stiles et Goldberger, 1910]

(Figs. 21–24)

Specific Characters:

True ventral atrium absent; pharynx of calicophoron type; terminal genitalium papillogenitalis type (genital atrium provided with tegumental papillae on its wall; well developed genital sphincter); acetabulum of calicophoron type.

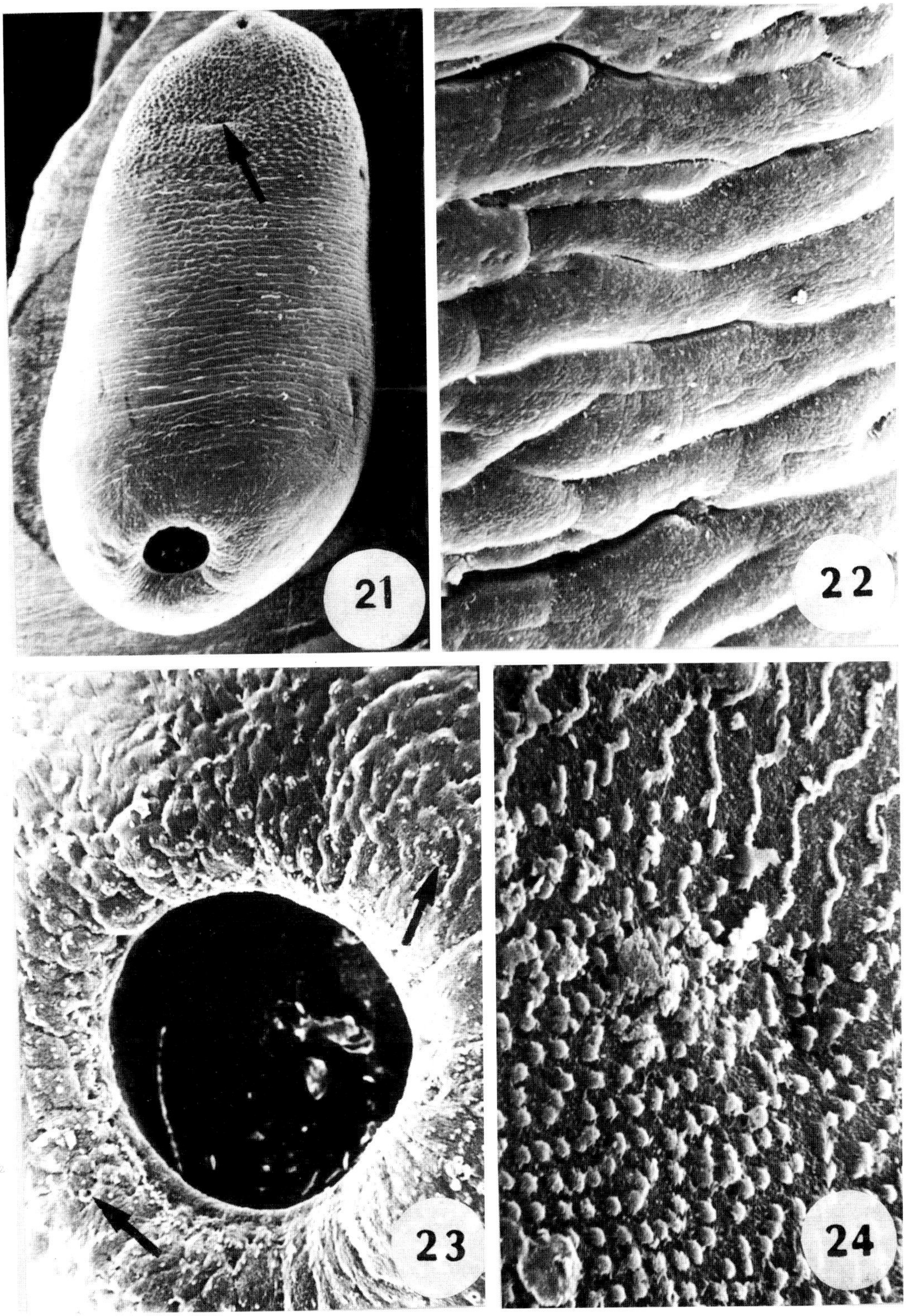

Figs. 21–24. *Calicophoron papillosum*.
21: Whole worm, ventral view. Note the aggregation of minute papillae surrounding the genital pore opening (arrow). × 20
22: Dorsal surface of body, showing wrinkles or tegumental folds.
23: Acetabular aperture, showing radial corrugations of the rim and minute pits (arrows) around it. × 120
24: Domed papillae and ridges at the base of genital papilla. × 200

Species: *Calicophoron shillongensis* Roy et Tandon, 1995

(Figs. 25–28)

Specific characters:

Pharynx of calicophoron type; terminal genitalium of shillongensis type (deep and enormous ventral atrium, weakly developed genital papilla and sphincter papilla); acetabulum of cotylophoron type (d.e.c.m. and v.e.c.m. clearly separated by an obliquely running and longitudinally branched muscle band).

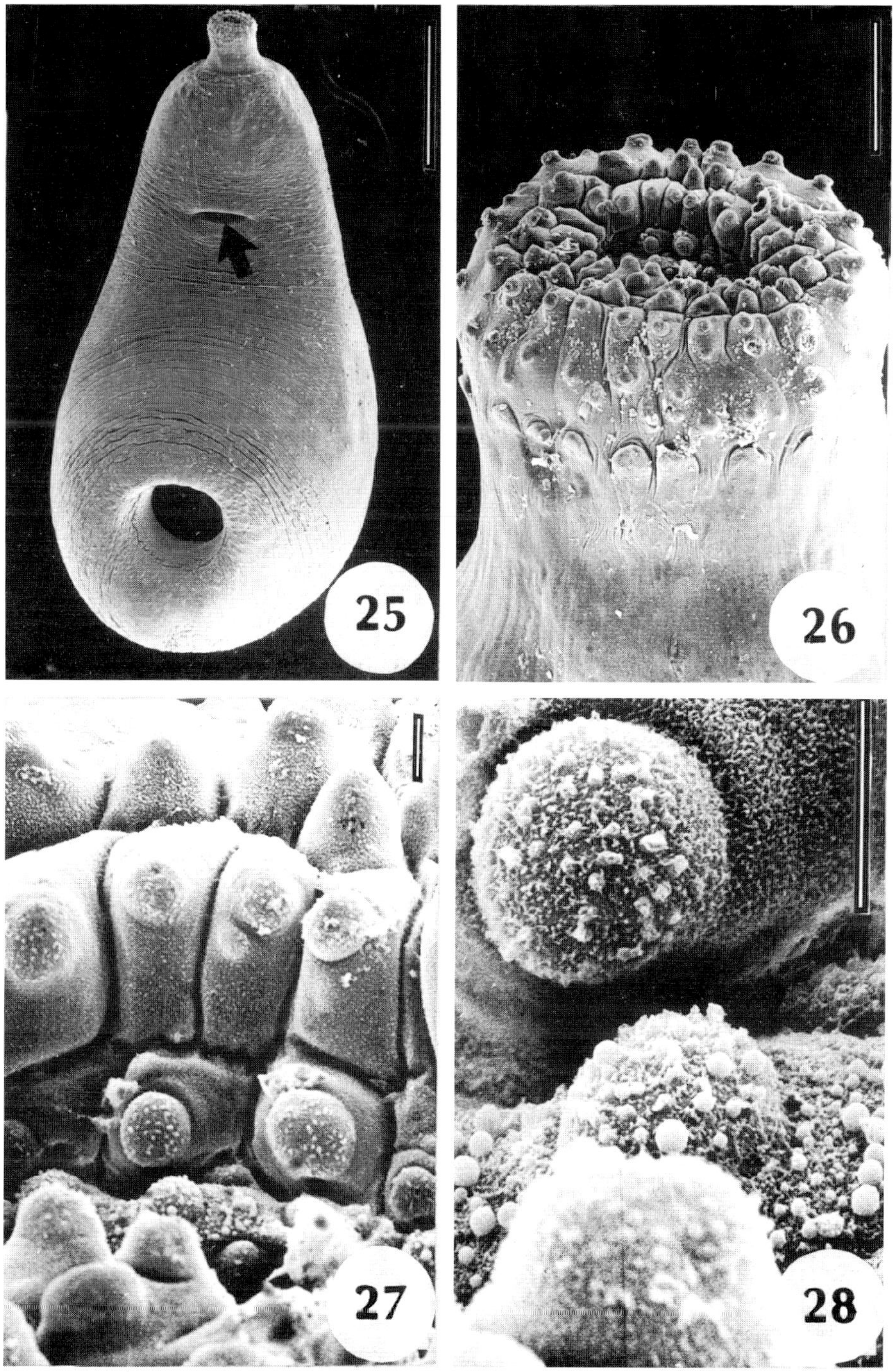

Figs. 25–28. *Calicophoron shillongensis*.
25: Whole worm, ventral view. Extensive genital atrium is visible (arrow). × 22
26: Anterior end of the body, showing characteristic arrangement of oral papillae. × 200
27: Ciliated round papillae in plate-like structures arranged in the inner wall of pharynx. × 940
28: Enlarged view of ciliated round papillae. × 2600

Genus : *Explanatum* (Fukui, 1929) Eduardo, 1984
Host : *Bos indicus*, *Bubalus bubalis*
Habitat : Bile duct, occasionally rumen and intestine
Species : *Explanatum explanatum* (Creplin, 1847) Fukui, 1929
[Syn. *Paramphistomum fraternum* Stiles et Goldberger, 1910
Paramphistomum siamense Stiles et Goldberger, 1910]

(Figs. 29–34)

Specific characters:

Body large, acetabulum relatively very large, far apart from pharynx; pharynx of explanatum type (smooth internal surface); caeca almost straight; terminal genitalium of explanatum type (genital sphincter absent, sphincter papilla present, radial musculature of genital atrium well developed), pars musculosa very short and weakly developed; acetabulum of explanatum type (d.e.c.m. divided into two parts, d.e.c.m. 1 and d.e.c.m. 2; former very strongly developed; limit towards d.e.c.m. 2 very sharp and clear).

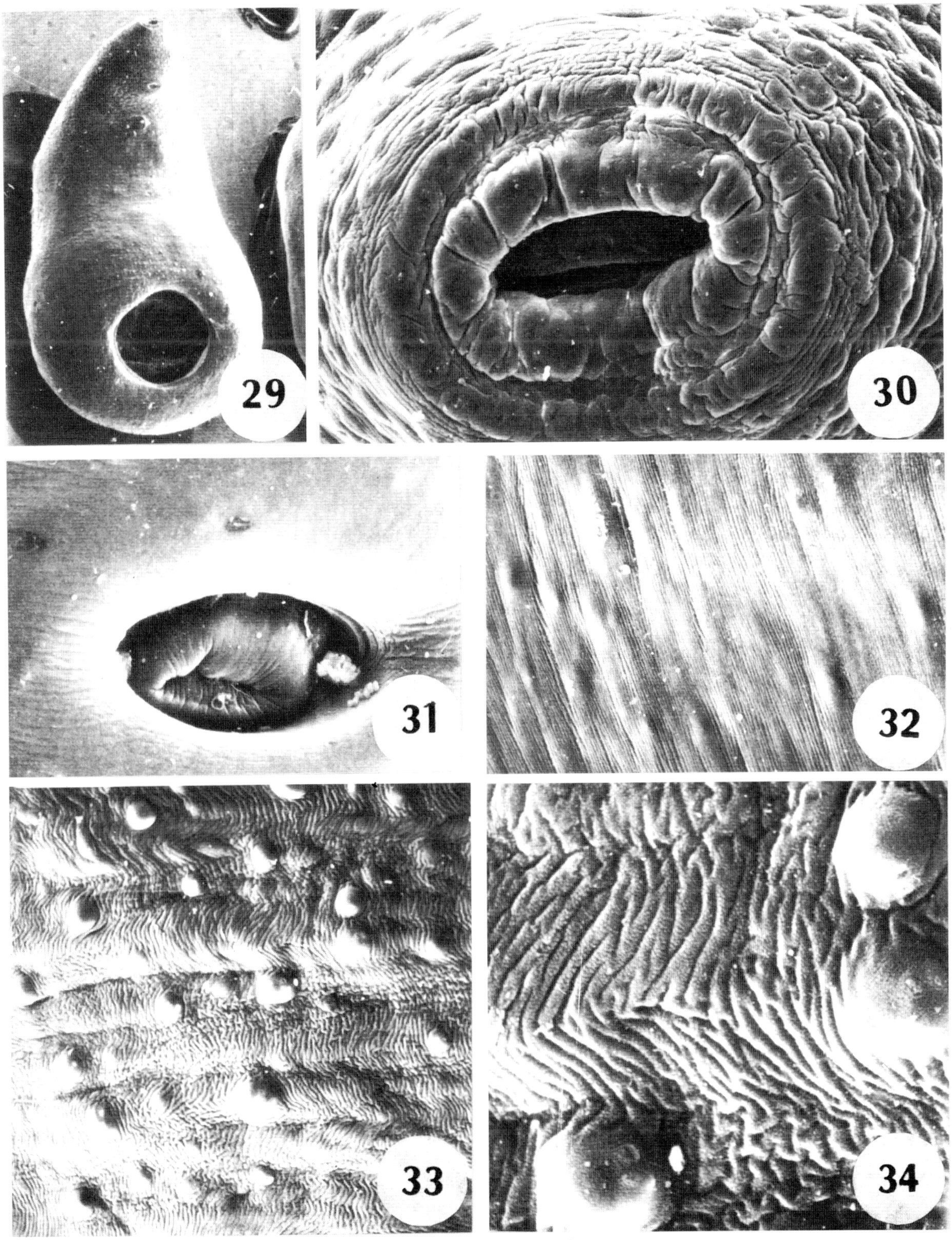

Figs. 29–34. *Explanatum explanatum.*
29: Whole worm, ventral view. Huge size of the acetabulum is very much characteristic for the genus. × 20
30: Oral aperture, top view. × 130
31: Genital pore region. × 160
32: Tegument of dorsal surface, showing minute tuberculation. × 660
33: Tegument of ventral surface. × 660
34: A portion of the enlarged ventral surface, showing fine wrinkles and domed smooth papillae. × 1800

Genus : *Orthocoelium* (Stiles et Goldberger, 1910) Price et McIntosh, 1953
Host : *Bos indicus*, *Ovis aries*, *Capra hircus*
Habitat : Rumen
Species : *Orthocoelium orthocoelium* (Fischoeder, 1901) Price et McIntosh, 1953

(Figs. 35–37)

Specific characters:

Pharynx of orthocoelium type (presence of a group of circular muscle units near anterior end forming anterior pharyngeal sphincter); oesophagus long with posterior sphincter; caeca straight, do not cross the dorsomedian line; terminal genitalium of orthocoelium type (thick genital papilla, well developed genital sphincter, sphincter papilla present); acetabulum of streptocoelium type (d.e.c.m. and v.e.c.m. units almost equal in size, dorsal interior circular muscles (d.i.c.m.) and ventral interior circular muscles (v.i.c.m.) units more in number than exterior ones and relatively strongly developed, interior circular series forming an arc-shaped curve).

Species : *Orthocoelium dicranocoelium* (Fischoeder, 1901) Yamaguti, 1971
[Syn. *Paramphistomum orthocoelium* Fischoeder, 1901
Ceylonocotyle orthocoelium Näsmark, 1937
C. tamilensis Gupta et Bakshi in Gupta and Nakhasi, 1977
Paramphistomum spinicephalus Tandon, 1955
Orthocoelium saccocoelium Sey, 1980]

(Fig. 38)

Specific characters:

Pharynx of dicranocoelium type (lip sphincter present, pharyngeal sacs absent, middle circular muscle layer absent); Oesophageal bulb present; caeca do not cross the dorsomedian line; terminal genitalium of gracile type (genital sphincter and sphincter papilla absent, genital folds lacking tegumental papillae); acetabulum streptocoelium type.

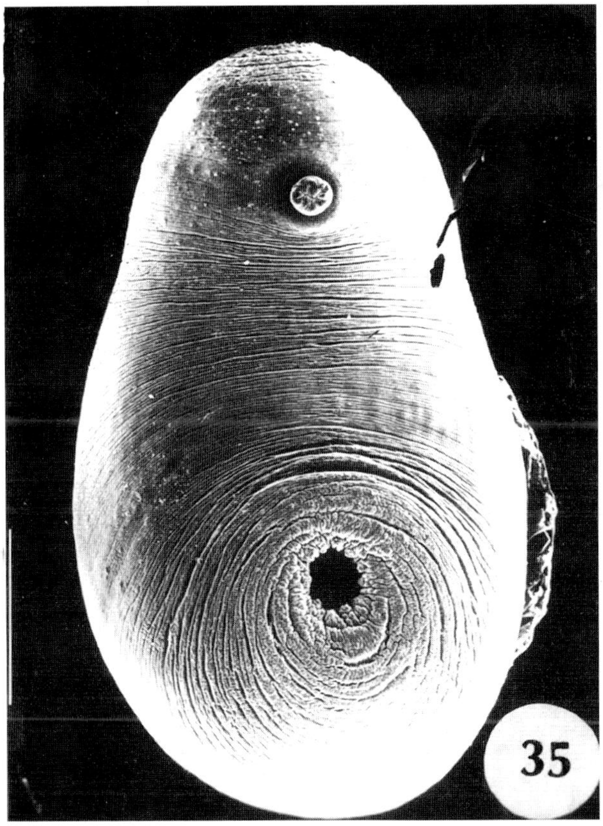

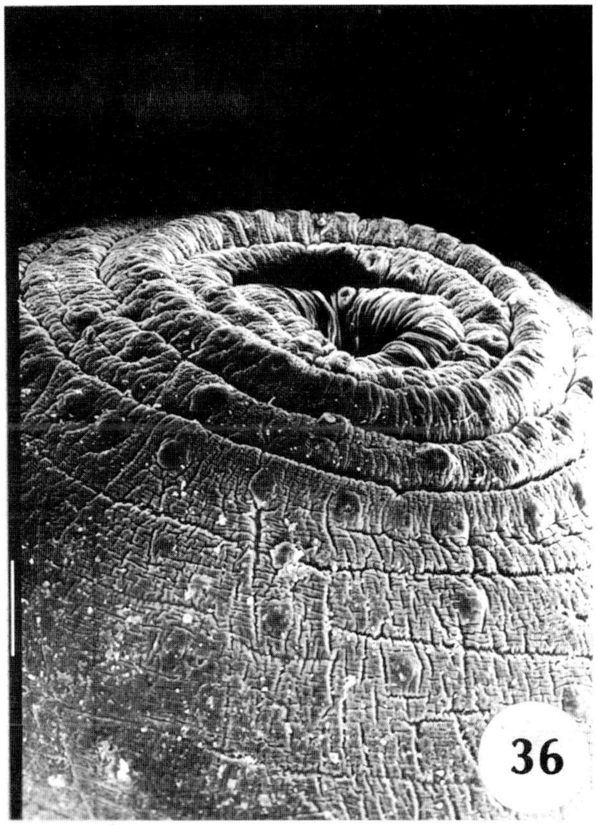

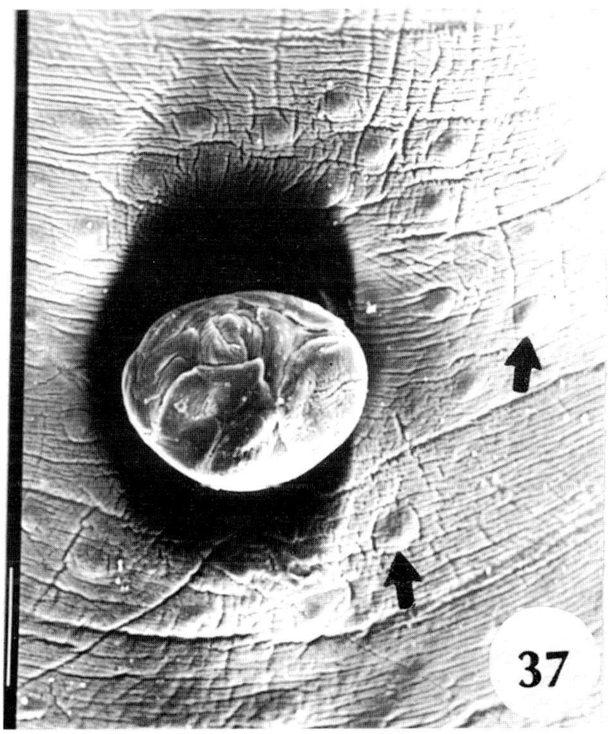

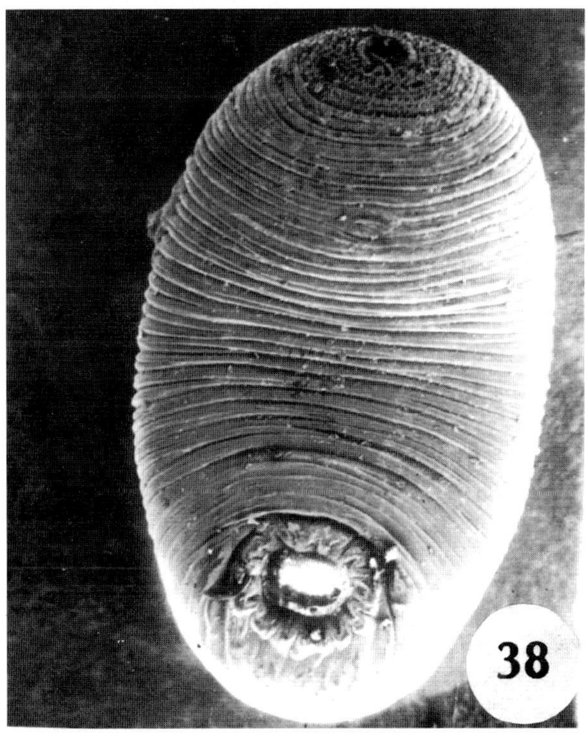

Figs. 35–37. *Orthocoelium orthocoelium*.
35: Whole worm, ventral view. Note the radial foldings of acetabular rim. × 22
36: Circum-oral region, showing button-shaped papillae in concentric rings. × 130
37: Terminal genitalium, showing everted genital papilla and minute domed papillae (arrows) on its surrounding tegument.× 160

Fig. 38. *Orthocoelium dicranocoelium*. Ventral view. Radial corrugation of the acetabular rim is clear. × 30

Species: *Orthocoelium scoliocoelium* (Fischoeder, 1904) Yamaguti, 1971
[Syn. *Paramphistomum scoliocoelium* Fischoeder, 1904
Cotylophoron ovatum Harshey, 1934]

(Figs. 39, 40, 45, 46)

Specific characters:

Pharynx of dicranocoelium type; oesophageal bulb present; caeca do not cross dorsomedian line; terminal genitalium of scoliocoelium type (genital sphincter and sphincter papilla present); acetabulum of streptocoelium type.

Species: *Orthocoelium dawesi* (Gupta, 1958) Yamaguti, 1971
[Syn. *Ceylonocotyle dawesi* Gupta, 1958]

(Figs. 41, 42)

Specific characters:

Pharynx of dicranocoelium type; oesophageal bulb present; caeca do not cross dorsomedian line; terminal genitalium of dawesi type (genital sphincter present, sphincter papilla absent); acetabulum of streptocoelium type.

Species: *Orthocoelium streptocoelium* (Fischoeder, 1901) Yamaguti, 1971
[Syn. *Paramphistomum streptocoelium* Fischoeder, 1901]

(Figs. 43, 44)

Specific characters:

Pharynx of calicophoron type; lip sphincter of pharynx and oesophageal bulb absent, posterior oesophageal sphincter present; caeca do not cross dorsomedian line; terminal genitalium of streptocoelium type (genital papilla thick, strongly developed sphincter papilla connected to well developed genital sphincter, genital fold lacks tegumental papillae); acetabulum of streptocoelium type.

Figs. 39, 40, 45. *Orthocoelium scoliocoelium.*
39: Whole worm, ventral view. × 30
40: Oral opening encircled by concentric tegumental folds studded with papillae. × 200

Figs. 41–42. *O. dawesi.*
41: General body surface. × 720
42: Whole worm in ventral view. × 30

Figs. 43–44. *O. streptocoelium.*
43: Tegument of the dorsal surface. × 120
44: Whole worm in ventral view. × 30

Fig. 45. *O. Scoliocoelium.* Ventral surface, showing deep folds of tegument and scattered minute papillae. × 660

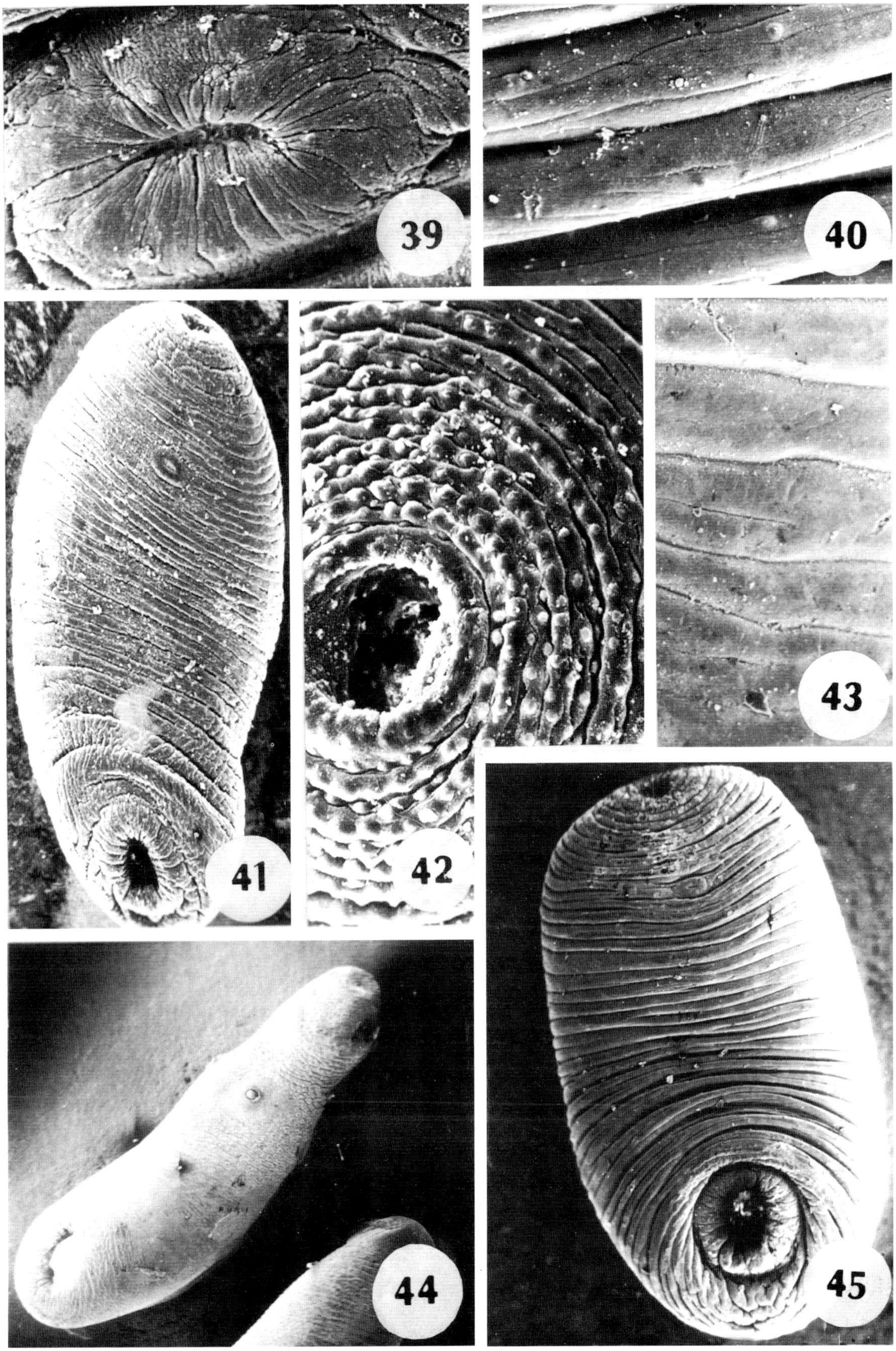
39
40
41
42
43
44
45

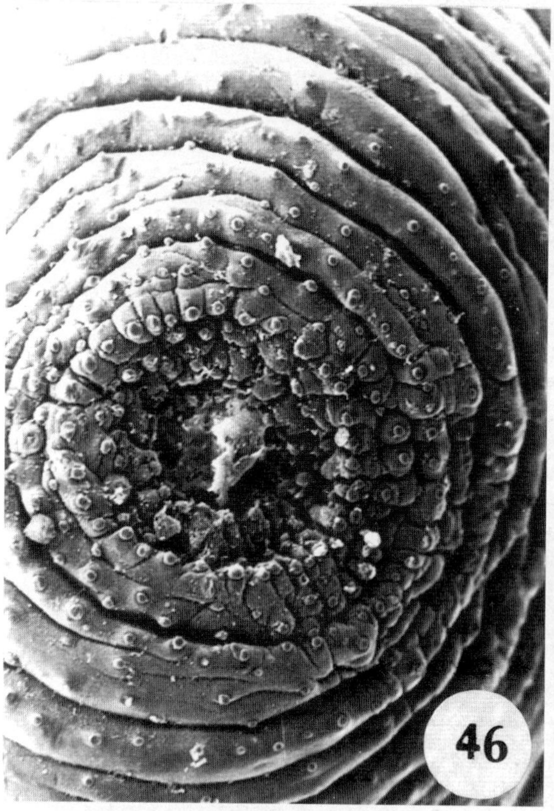

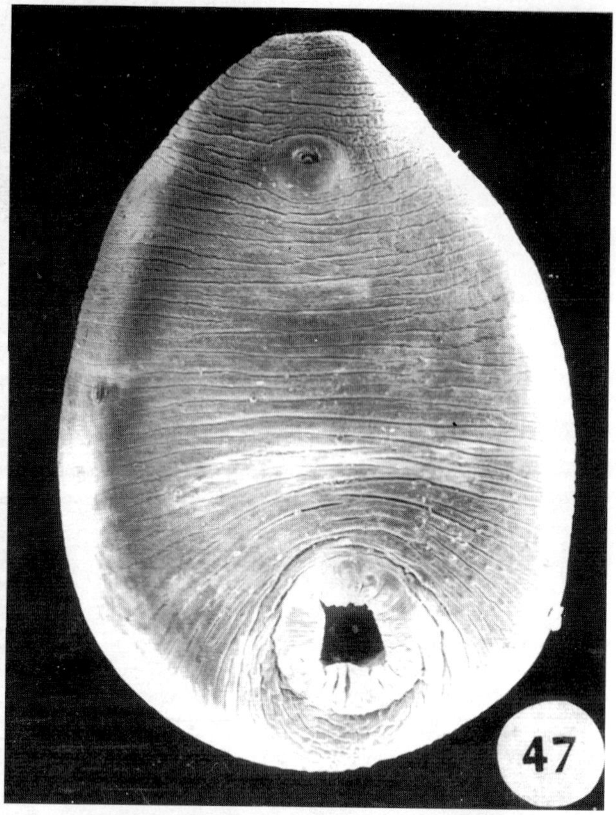

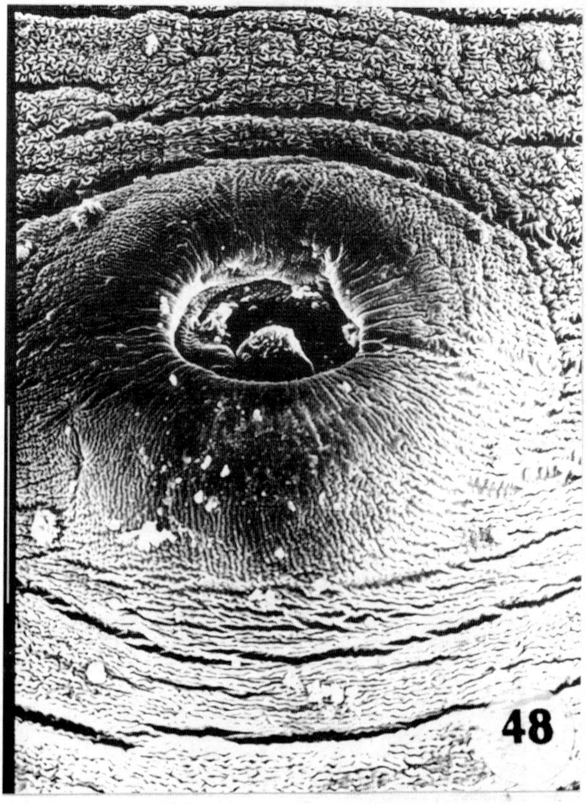

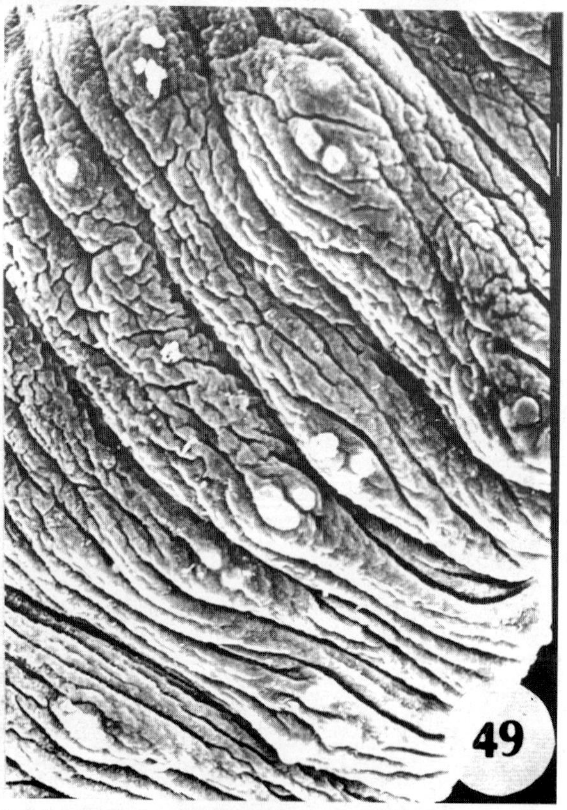

Fig. 46. *Orthocoelium scoliocoelium.* Oral sucker, top view, showing arrangement of papillae in circular ridges. × 200

Figs. 47–49. *O. parvipapillatum.*
47: Whole worm, ventral view. × 36
48: Region of genital opening. Note the fine tegumental folds but no papillae. × 260
49: Rim of acetabulum, showing tiny grouped papillae in between the radial folds. × 720

Species: *Orthocoelium parvipapillatum* (Stiles et Goldberger, 1910) Eduardo, 1985

(Figs. 47–49)

Specific characters:

Pharynx of dicranocoelium type; oesophageal bulb present, caeca do not cross dorsomedian line; terminal genitalium of parvipapillatum type (genital sphincter and sphincter papilla absent, genital fold provided with tegumental papillae); acetabulum of streptocoelium type.

Genus : *Leiperocotyle* Eduardo, 1980
Hosts : *Bos indicus*, *Bubalus bubalis*
Habitat : Rumen
Species : *Leiperocotyle meghalayensis* Roy et Tandon, 1992

(Figs. 50–53)

Specific characters:

Laurer's canal not crossing excretory vesicle or duct; pharynx of calicophoron type; oesophageal bulb present; blind intestinal caeca terminating ventrally; terminal genitalium cotylophoron type (genital atrium forms genital sucker having clear delimiting membrane against tissues of body); acetabulum of streptocoelium type.

Figs. 50–53. *Leiperocotyle meghalayensis*.
50: Whole worm, ventral view. × 36
51: Anterior region showing tegumental smooth and domed papillae around the oral aperture and genital opening (arrow). × 94
52: Enlarged view of acetabular region. × 94
53: Clustered arrangement of papillae in between the radial tegumental ridges of the acetabular rim. × 780

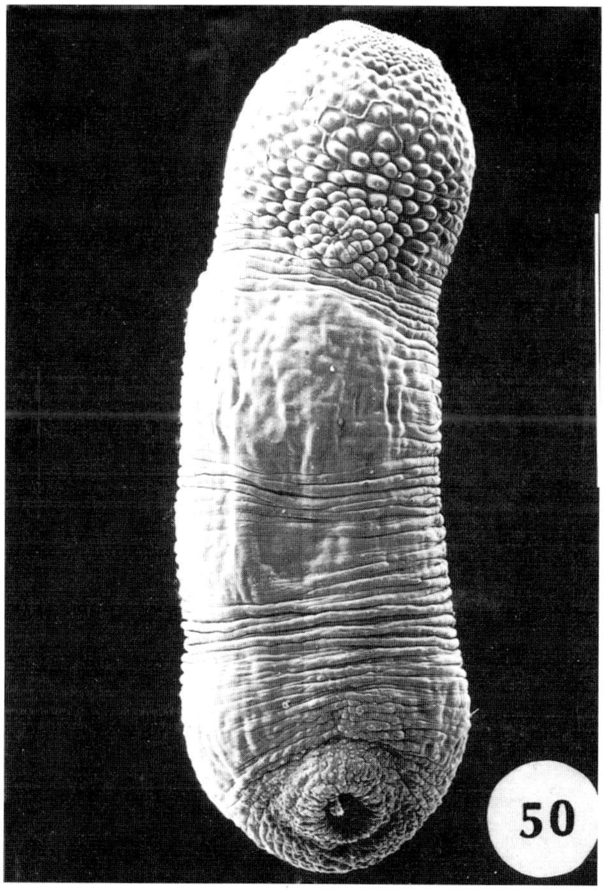

50

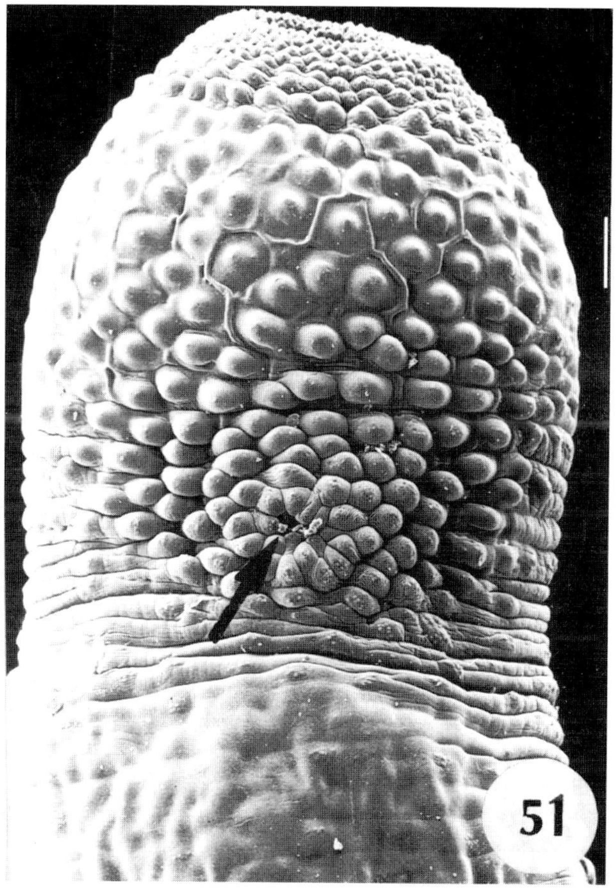

51

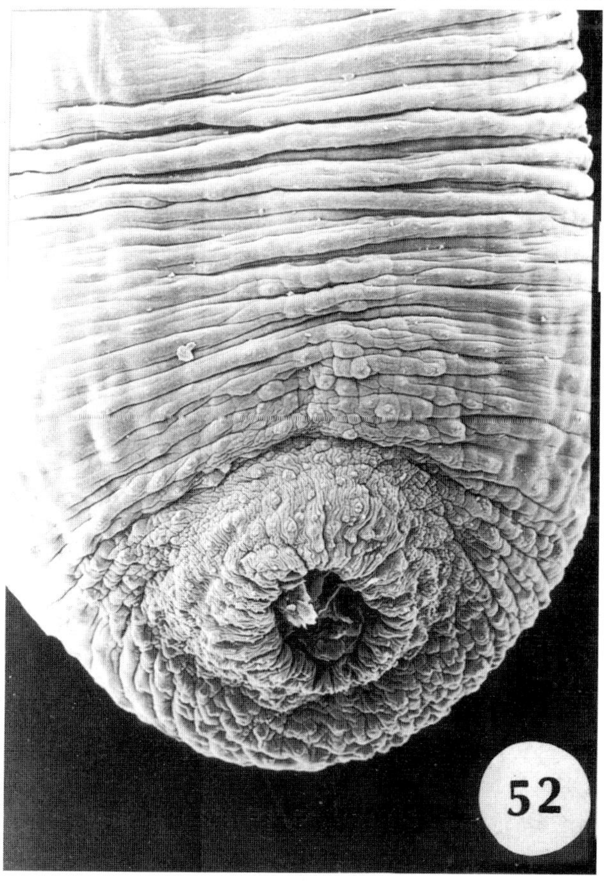

52

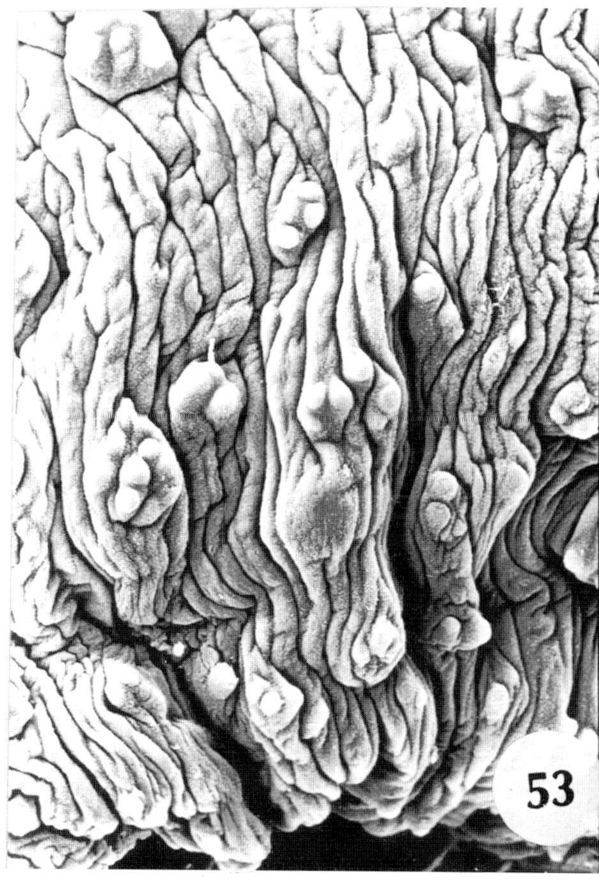

53

Genus : *Olveria* Thapar et Sinha, 1945
Host : *Bos indicus*, *Bubalus bubalis*
Habitat : Rumen
Species : *Olveria indica* Thapar et Sinha, 1945

(Figs. 54–58)

Specific characters:

Pharynx with two pouches, triangular in shape; oesophagus 'J' shaped, caeca with two coils; terminal genitalium of papillogenitalium type; acetabulum of stichorchis type (d.e.c.m. and v.e.c.m. units very close to each other at the margin of acetabulum, interior circular muscles (i.c.m.) spread over a large part of inner acetabular periphery, numerous lymphatic ramifications present in between radial muscle fibres of acetabular tissue).

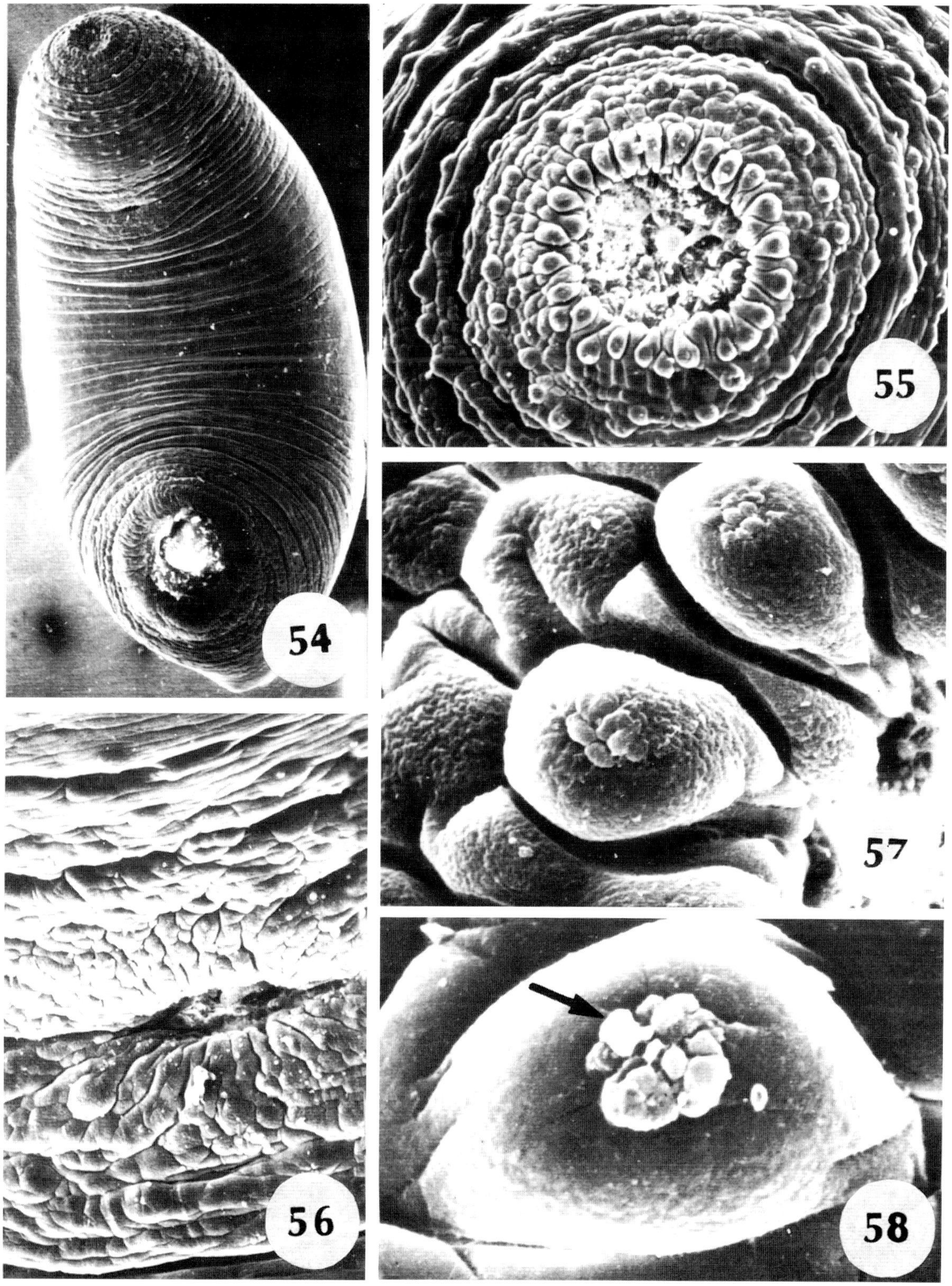

Figs. 54–58. *Olveria indica*.
54: Whole worm, ventral view. × 30
55: Tegumental architecture of the circum-oral region and studded with modular elevations. × 120
56: Tegumental corrugations in the region surrounding the genital pore and studded with nodular elevations. × 660
57: A magnified view of the oral rim, showing arrangement of petaloid papillae and tegumental foldings. × 2000
58: Closer view of a single circum-oral petaloid elevation with clustered papillae at the top (arrow). × 4000

Species: *Olveria bosi* Tandon, 1951

(Figs. 59–63)

Specific characters:

Pharynx with two pouches, round in shape; oesophagus ‘J’ shaped; caeca with three loops, terminating blindly in front of acetabulum and curved inward at their posterior extremities, lying one behind the other.

Figs. 59–63. *Olveria bosi*.
59: Whole worm, ventral view. × 36
60: Anterior region of body. Note the oral aperture free from any papillate structure. × 130
61: Oral aperture in top view, showing fine tegumental folding. The rim of the oral aperture is radially corrugated and inner wall of the pharynx is provided with spine-like papillae. × 720
62: A closer view of pharyngeal papillae. × 3000
63: Clustered smooth papillae at the genital opening. × 660

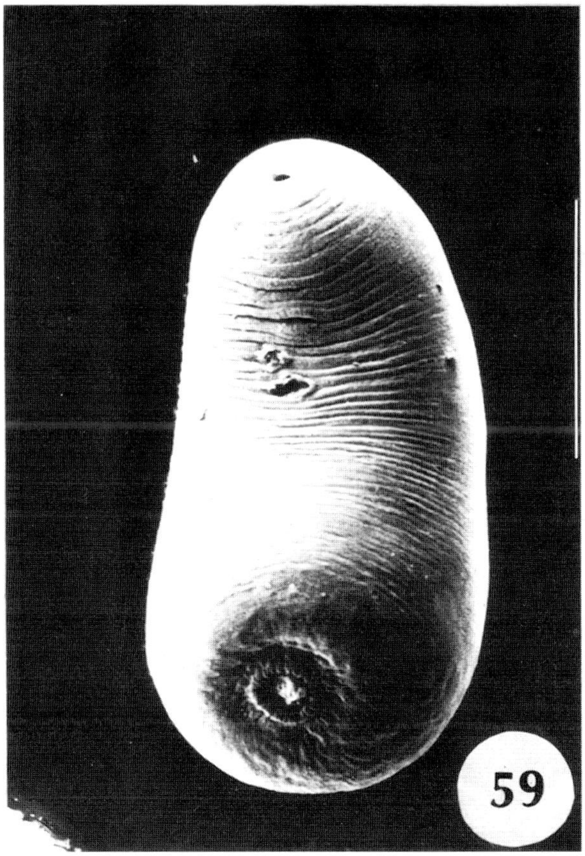
59

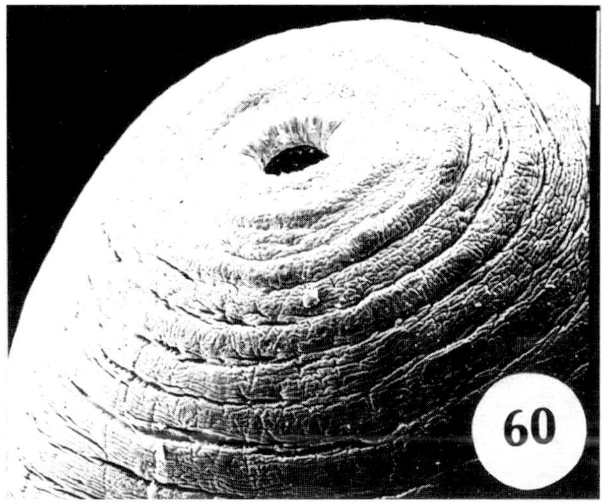
60

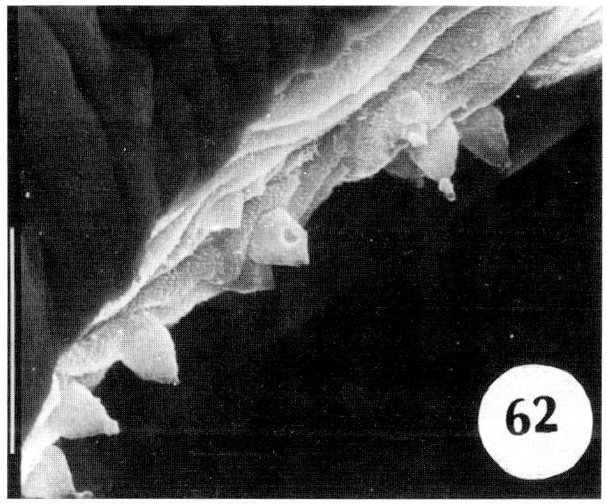
62

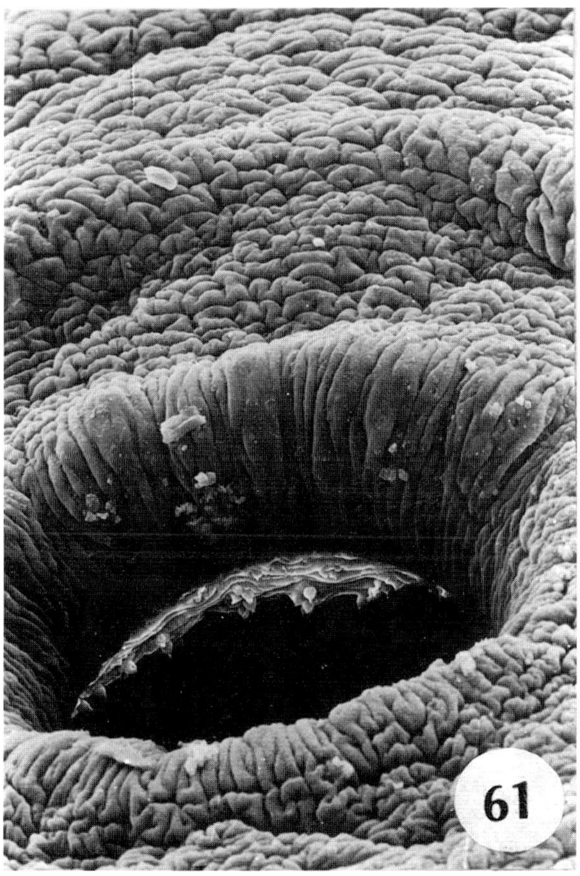
61

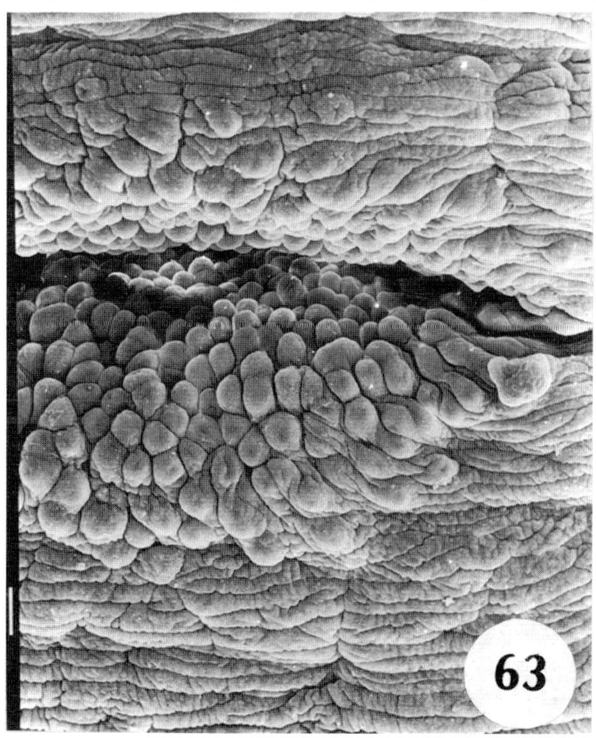
63

Genus : *Gastrodiscoides* Leiper, 1913
Host : *Sus scrofa domestica*
Habitat : Large intestine
Species : *Gastrodiscoides hominis* (Lewis et McConnell, 1876) Leiper, 1913
[Syn. *Gastrodiscus hominis* Fischoeder, 1902]

(Figs. 64–66)

Specific characters:

Pharynx of watsonius type (pharyngeal bulb and secondary pharyngeal sac present, middle circular layer with very strongly developed units); oesophageal bulb present; terminal genitalium with genital fold having domed papillae; genital pore at level of oesophagus; acetabulum of watsonius type (c.m. units more strongly developed in exterior series, smaller and uniform in size in middle part of sucker).

Genus : *Homalogaster* Poirier, 1883
Host : *Bos indicus*, *Bubalus bubalis*
Habitat : Intestine
Species : *Homalogaster paloniae* Poirier, 1883
[Syn. *Homalogaster poirier* Giard et Billet, 1892, in Railliet et al., 1914
Homalogaster philippinensis Stiles et Goldberger, 1910]

(Figs. 67–68)

Specific characters:

Pharynx of homalogaster type (pharyngeal bulb, secondary pharyngeal sacs present; anterior muscle units loosely packed without forming an anterior sphincter); terminal genitalium of homalogaster type (genital papilla large with swollen tip, well-developed circular, longitudinal and dorsoventral muscle fibres present beneath the area surrounding pores); acetabulum of homalogaster type (v.e.c.m. divided into two groups, interior series increasing in unit size away from sucker rim, exterior series having a few irregular enlarged units near sucker rim).

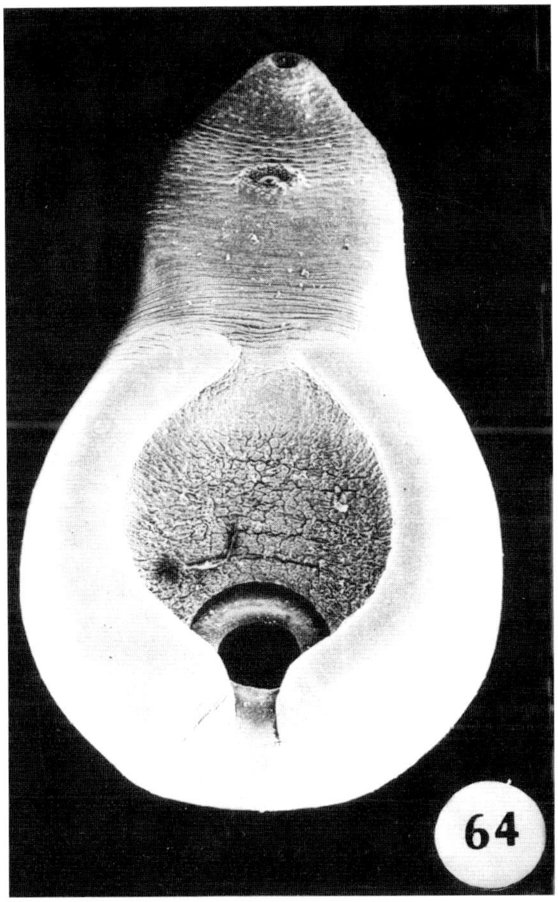

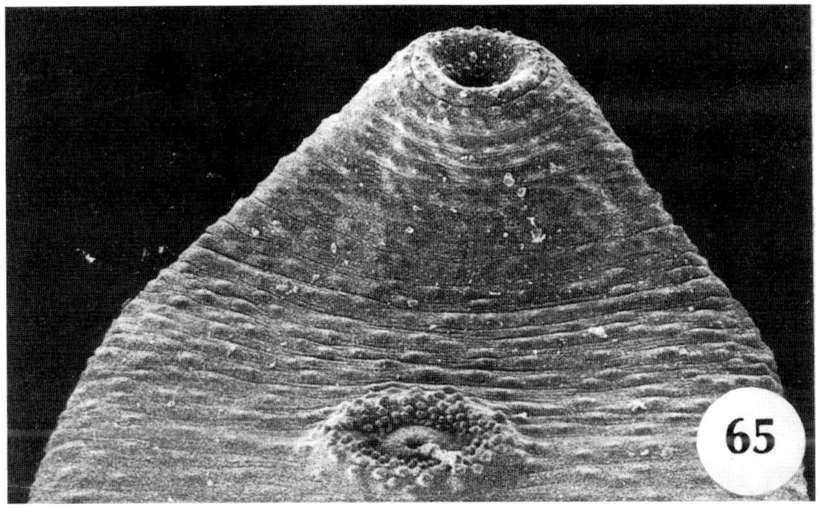

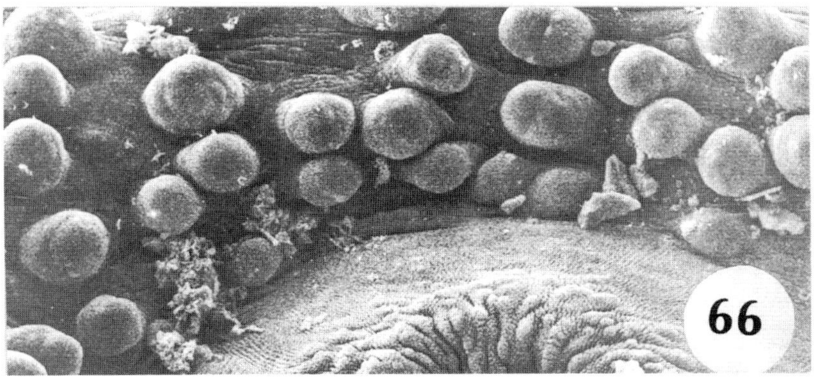

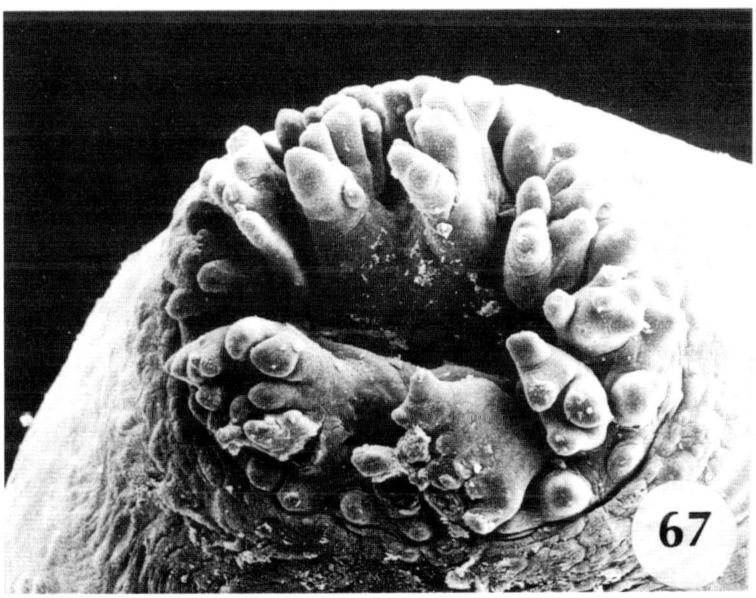

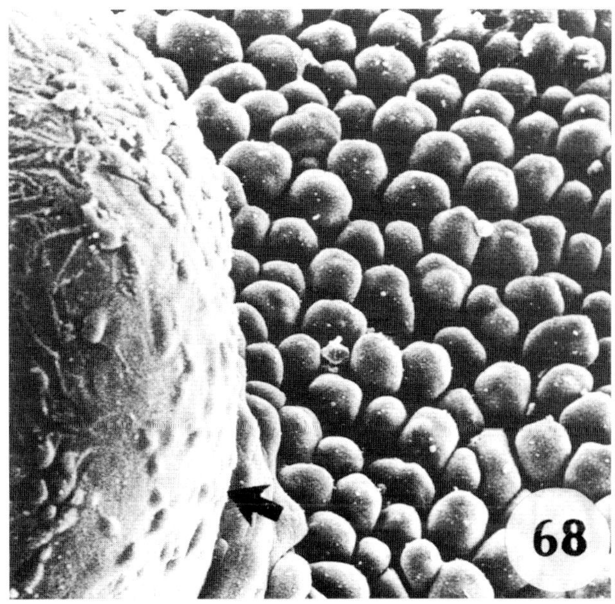

Figs. 64–66. *Gastrodiscoides hominis*.
64: Whole worm, ventral view. × 20
65: Anterior region of body, showing papillae in concentric rings surrounding the oral aperture and genital pore opening. × 60
66: Region of genital pore, showing conspicuous raised smooth papillae surrounding the pore. × 540

Figs. 67–68. *Homalogaster paloniae*.
67: Circum-oral region, showing branched oral papillae. These branched papillae are very much characteristic of the species. × 360
68: Tegumental surface of genital papilla (arrow) and its adjoining region in a closer view. × 540

Genus : *Fischoederius* Stiles et Goldberger, 1910
Host : *Bos indicus*, *Bubalus bubalis*, *Ovis aries*, *Capra hircus*
Habitat : Rumen
Species : *Fischoederius elongatus* (Poirier, 1883) Stiles et Goldberger, 1910

(Figs. 69–71)

Specific characters:

Ventral pouch present; pharynx of calicophoron type; caeca straight, terminate before middle of body; terminal genitalium lying ventrally inside ventral pouch at level posterior to pharynx, of elongatus type (genital papillae and median papillae provided with genital sphincter and ventral sphincter, tegumental papillae present only in median papillae); acetabulum of gastrothylax type (inner cavity of acetabulum basin shaped, d.e.c.m. and v.e.c.m. displaying very large number of units which exceeds that of units in d.i.c.m. and v.i.c.m.).

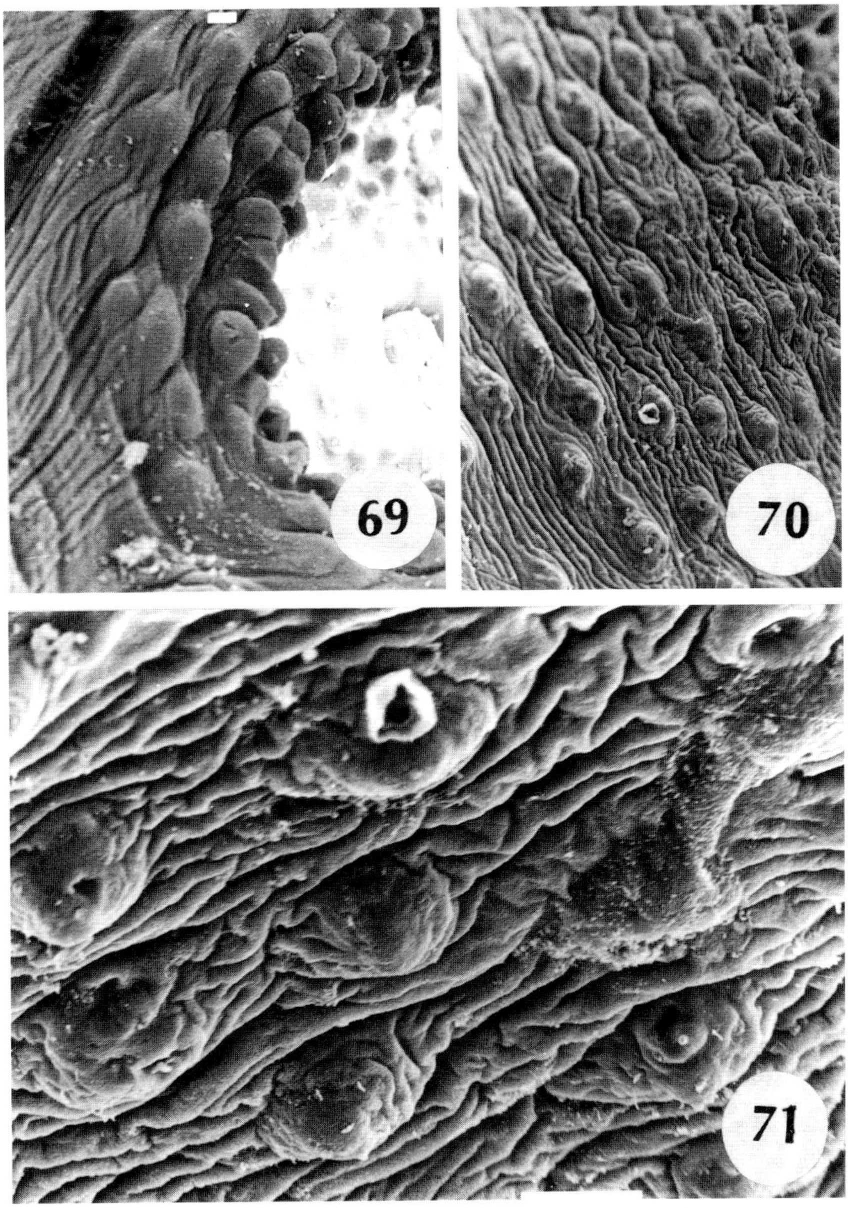

Figs. 69–71. *Fischoederius elongatus*.
69: Rim of oral sucker, showing smooth oral papillae. × 130
70: Tegumental papillae in the anterior region of body. × 540
71: Enlarged view of tegument, showing fine surface foldings and nature of papillae. × 1800

Species : *Fischoederius cobboldi* (Poirier, 1883) Stiles et Goldberger, 1910

(Figs. 72, 73)

Specific characters:

Ventral pouch present; pharynx of calicophoron type; 'S'-shaped oesophagus, caeca reaching up to anterior border of acetabulum; terminal genitalium of microbothrium type (genital sphincter considerable in size, well delimited from surrounding tissue, sphincter papillae fairly strongly developed); acetabulum of gastrothylax type.

Genus : *Gastrothylax* Poirier, 1883
Host : *Bos indicus*, *Bubalus bubalis*, *Ovis aries*, *Capra hircus*
Habitat : Rumen
Species : *Gastrothylax crumenifer* (Creplin, 1947) Poirier, 1883

(Figs. 74, 75)

Specific characters:

Ventral pouch present; pharynx of calicophoron type; long, wavy intestinal caeca reaching up to anterior level of testes; terminal genitalium of gracile type (with well developed genital papilla); acetabulum of gastrothylax type.

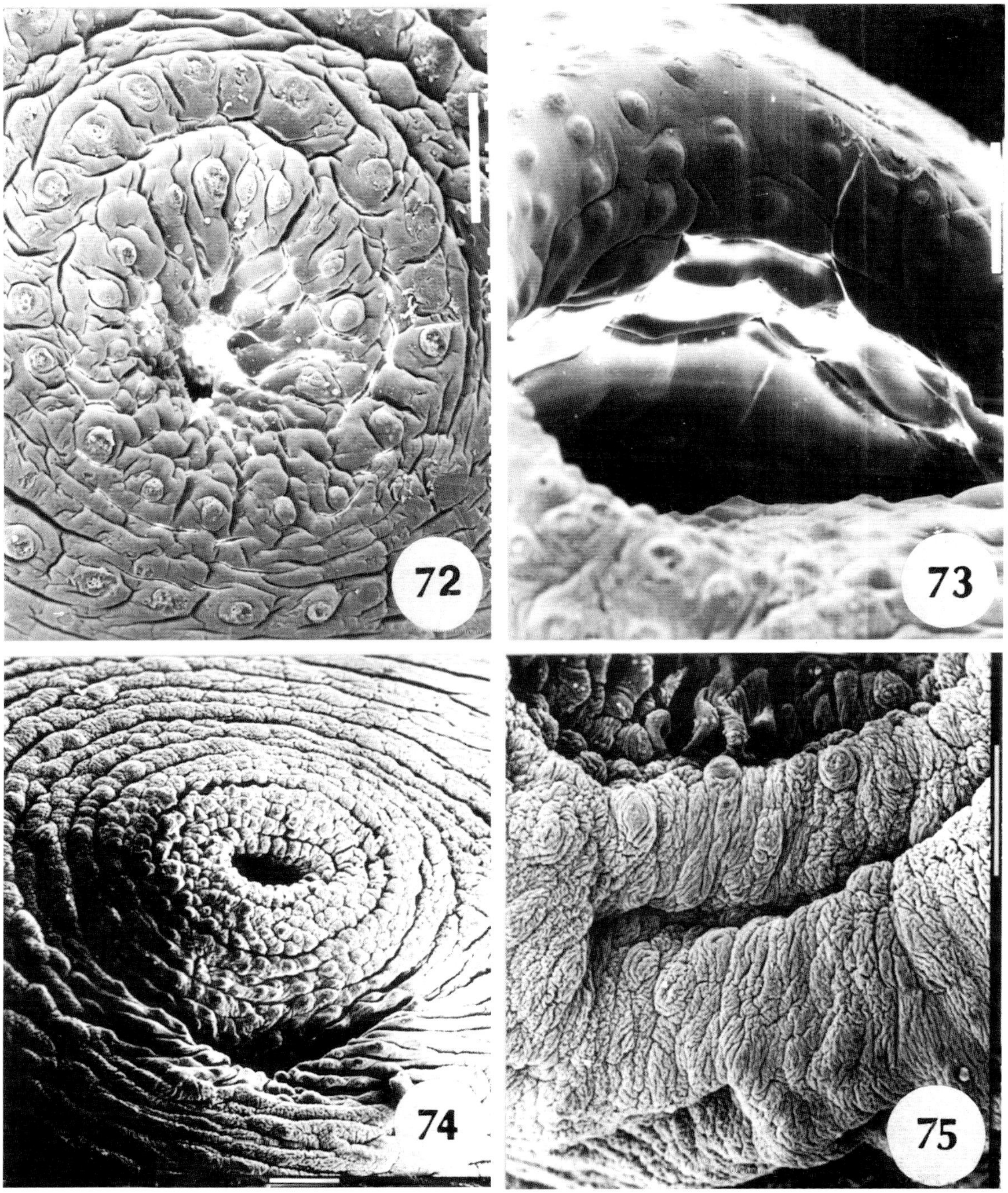

Figs. 72, 73. *Fischoederius cobboldi*.
72: Oral aperture, top view, showing arrangement of oral papillae around the mouth. × 200
73: Inner wall of oral aperture. × 600

Figs. 74, 75. *Gastrothylax crumenifer*.
74: Anterior end of body, showing oral aperture and ventral pouch opening. × 60
75: Rim of acetabulum. × 1000

Genus : *Carmyerius* Stiles et Goldberger, 1910
Host : *Ovis aries*, *Capra hircus*
Habitat : Rumen
Species : *Carmyerius spatiosus* (Brandes, 1898) Stiles et Goldberger, 1910

(Figs. 76–80)

Specific characters:

Ventral pouch present; pharynx of calicophoron type; caeca straight, reaching up to posterior region of body; terminal genitalium of gracile type; acetabulum of gastrothylax type.

Figs. 76–80. *Carmyerius spatiosus.*
76: Whole worm, ventral view. × 22
77: A part of oral aperture (top view), showing the arrangement of ciliated oral papillae in two rows. × 1000
78: Opening of ventral pouch. Clustered, smooth papillae are evident at the rim of the pouch. × 660
79: A portion of the rim of acetabulum. Note the radial foldings of tegument and clustered papillae in between the folds. × 300
80: Inner wall of acetabulum, showing rough surfaced papillae. × 3000

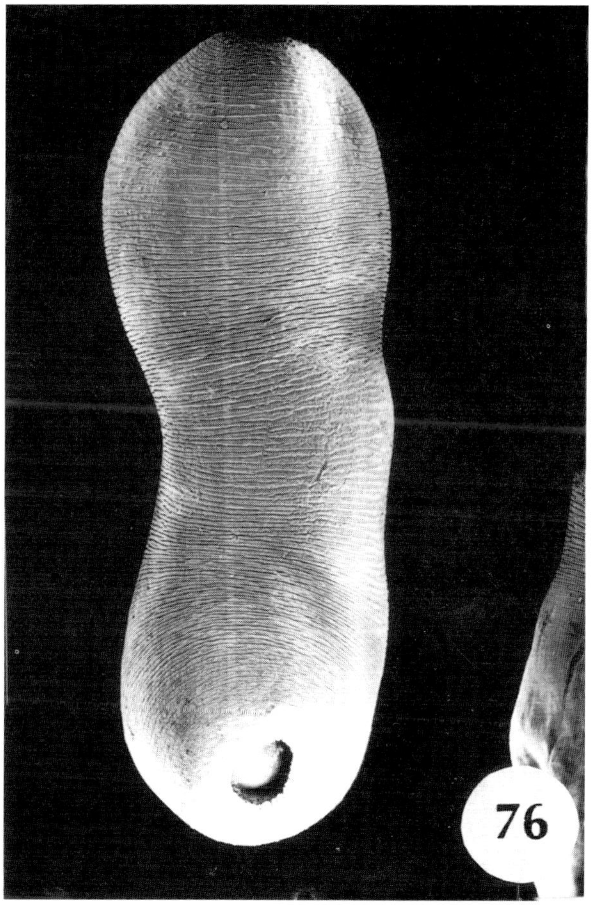
76

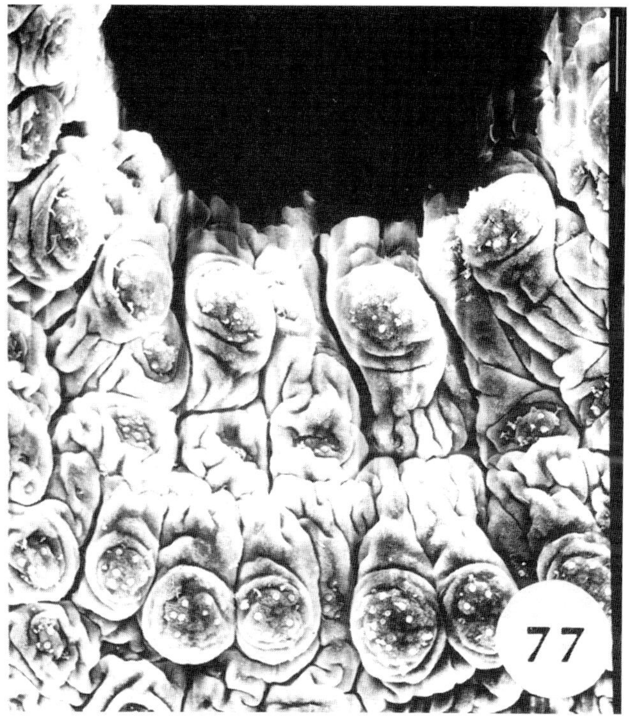
77

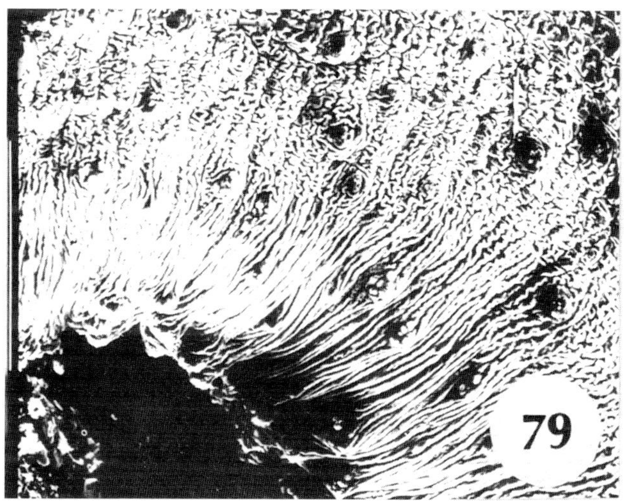
79

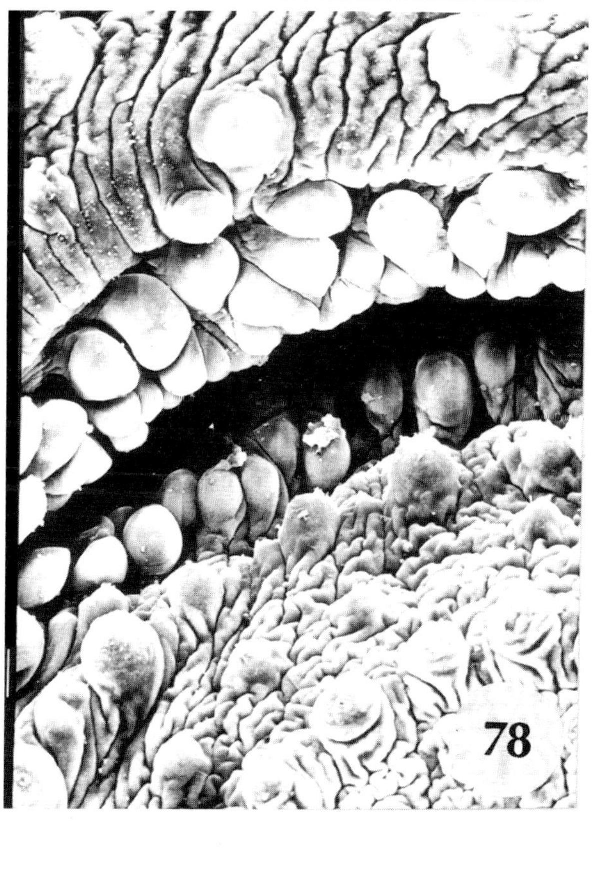
78

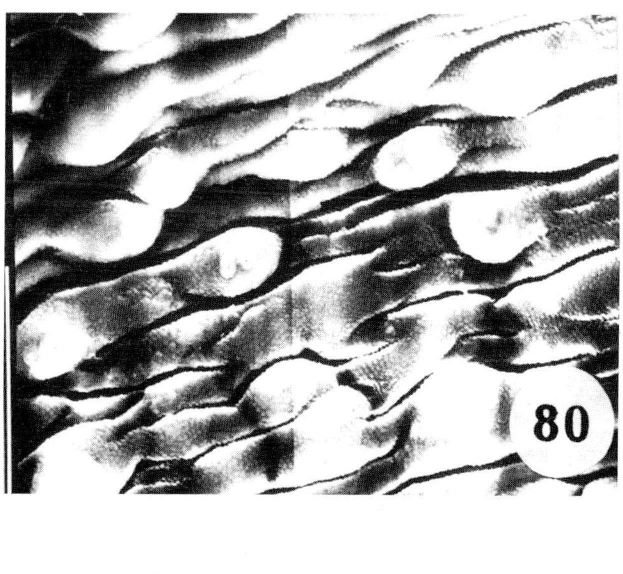
80

Genus : *Velasquezotrema* Eduardo et Javellana, 1987
Host : *Bos indicus*, *Bubalus bubalis*
Habitat : Rumen
Species : *Velasquezotrema tripurensis* Roy et Tandon, 1990

(Figs. 81–84)

Specific characters:

Ventral pouch extending up to middle of body; pharynx of calicophoron type, oesophageal sphincter present; terminal genitalium of tripurensis type (presence of dome-shaped papillae in the wall of protrusible ventral atrium, sphincter papillae weakly developed); acetabulum of gastrothylax type.

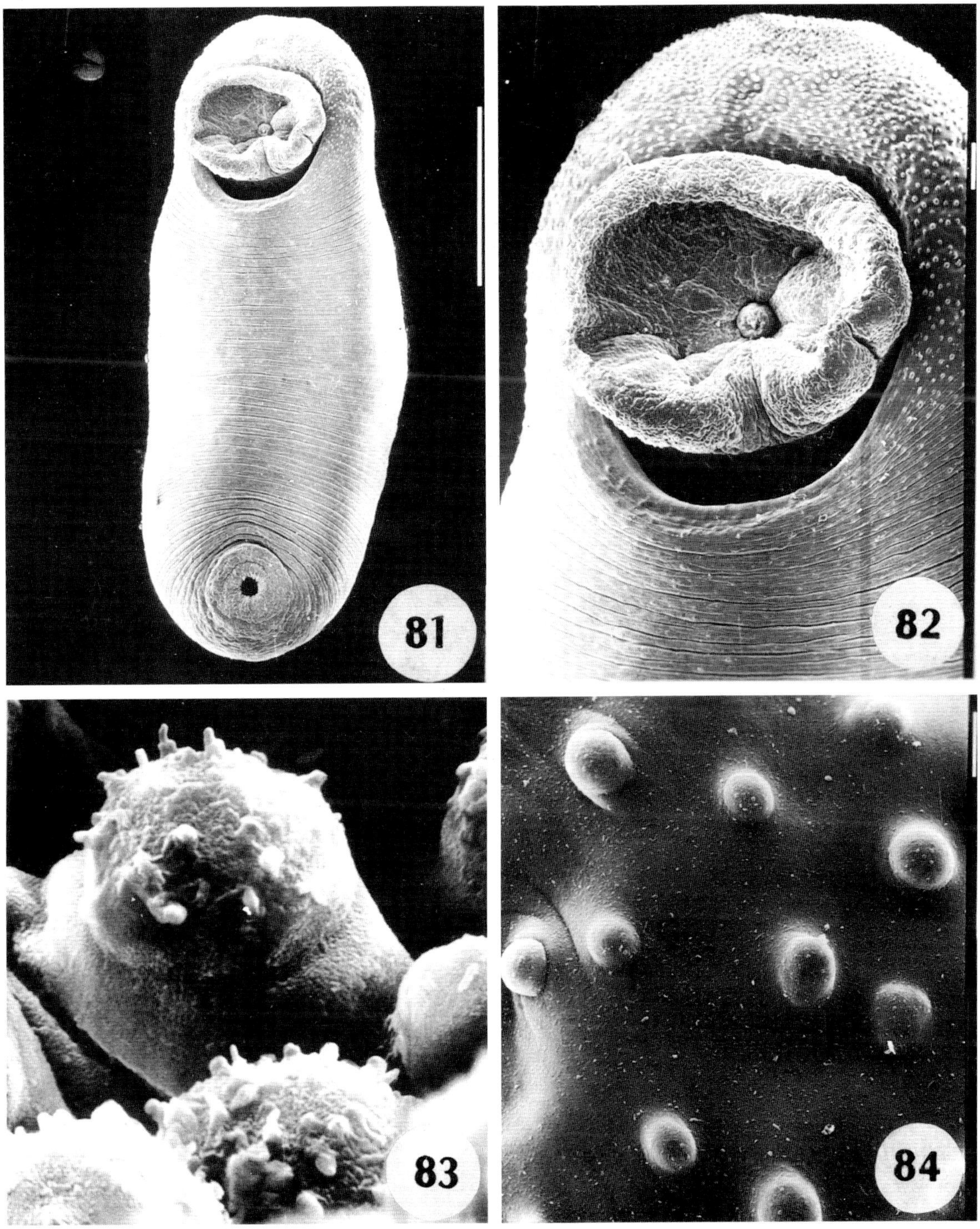

Figs. 81–84. *Velasquezotrema tripurensis*.
81: Whole worm in ventral view. The muscular disc is protruding out through the ventral pouch opening. × 26
82: Anterior region of body, showing the ejected muscular disc with papillae at the centre. × 72
83: A closer view of circum-oral papillae with many ciliary structures in each. × 4800
84: Smooth and round papillae on general body surface. × 1000

Genus : *Fasciola* Linnaeus, 1758
Host : *Bos indicus*, *Bubalus bubalis*, *Ovis aries*, *Capra hircus*
Habitat : Bile duct
Species : *Fasciola gigantica* Cobbold, 1858
[Syn. *Fasciola indica* Varma, 1953]

(Figs. 85–90)

Specific characters:

Cephalic cone relatively short; caeca branched externally; testes extensively branched, ovary branched, uterus forming rosette-like clusters of coils between ovary and acetabulum; vitellaria filling up all available space between caecal ramifications laterally.

Figs. 85, 86. *Fasciola gigantica*.
85: Anterior region of body, ventral view. Oral sucker is free from any papillae but has strong musculature. × 250
86: Anterior region of body, dorsal view, showing dense spination. × 180

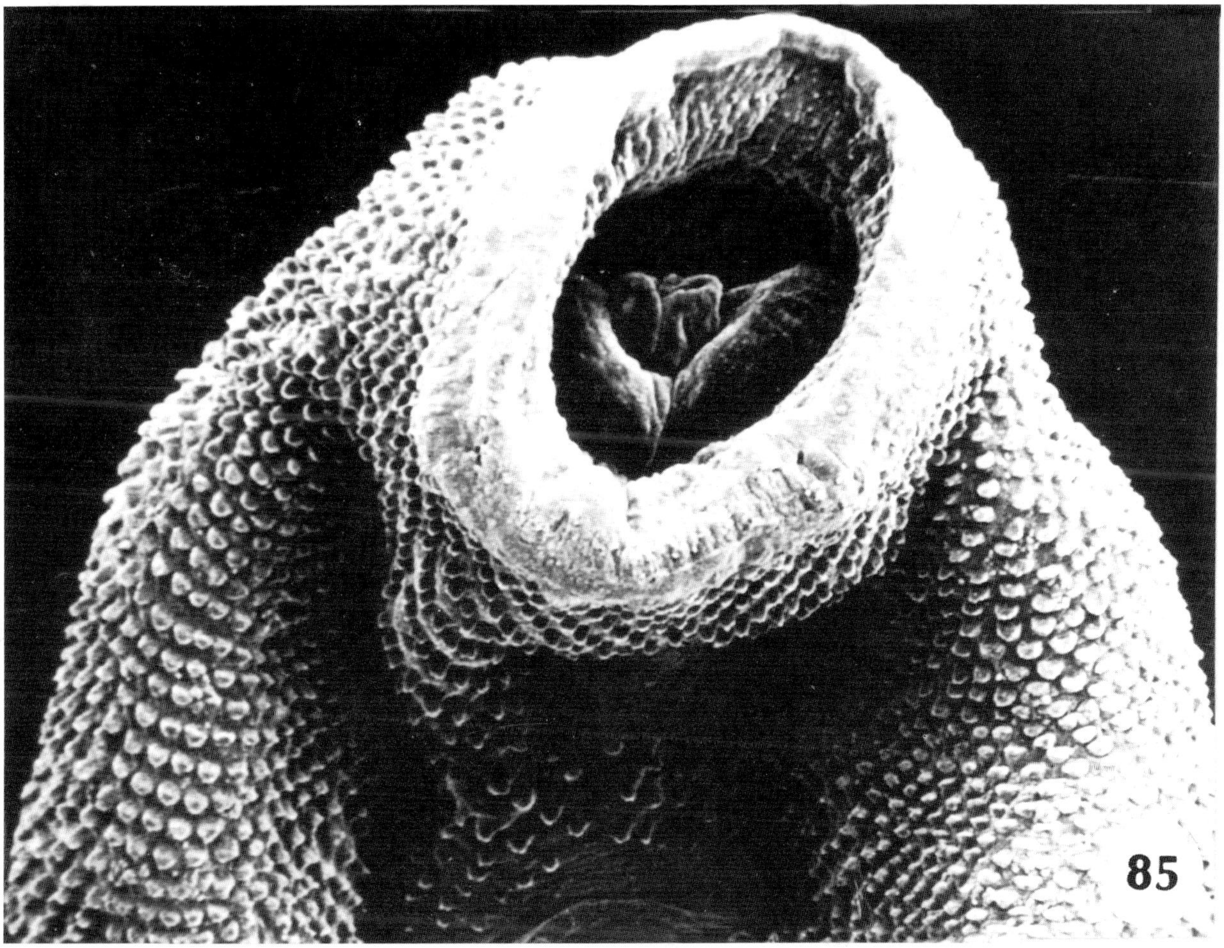
85

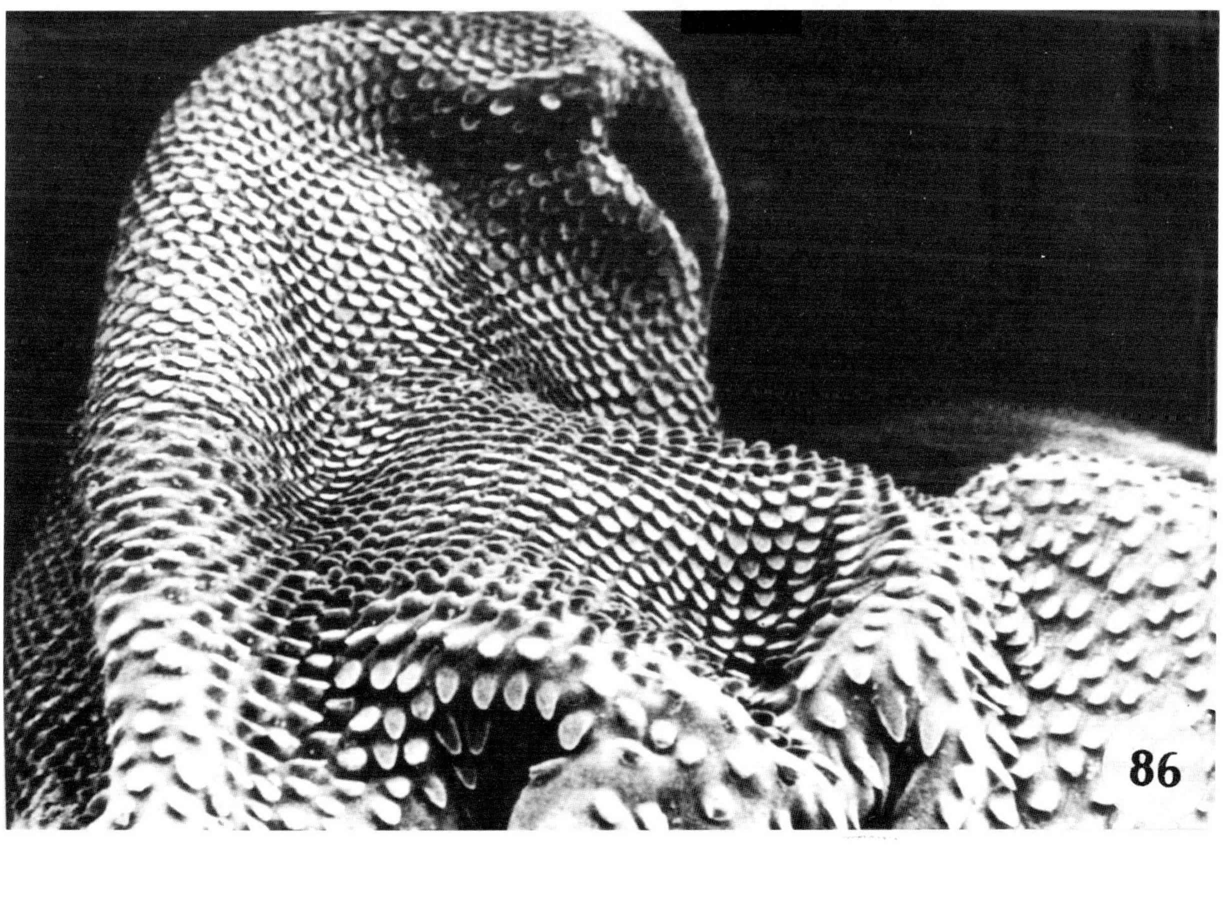
86

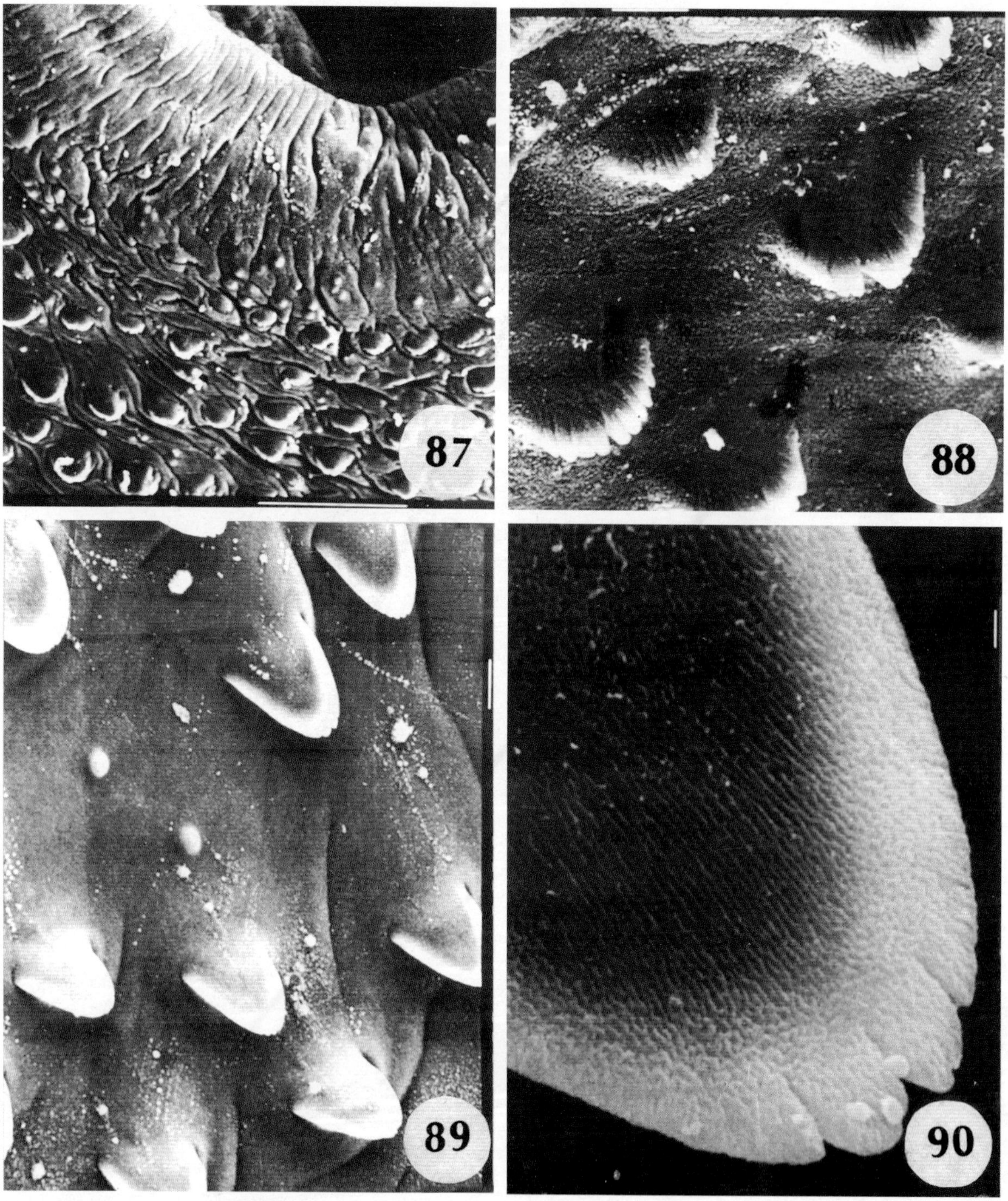

Figs. 87–90. *Fasciola gigantica*.
87: Rim of ventral sucker, with scales surrounding sucker. × 400
88: Enlarged view of scales. The tips of the scales are not smooth and are multi-pointed. × 1200
89: Spiny surface surrounding the oral sucker. × 800
90: One spine, enlarged, showing unsmooth surface and multi-pointed tip. × 6000

Genus : *Fasciolopsis* Looss, 1899
Host : *Sus scrofa domestica*
Habitat : Intestine
Species : *Fasciolopsis buski* (Lankester, 1857) Looss, 1899
[Syn. *Distoma crassum* Cobbold, 1860
Distoma rathouisi Poirier, 1887
Fasciolopsis fulleborni Roden Waldt, 1909
Fasciolopsis goddardi Ward, 1909
Fasciolopsis spinifera Brown, 1917]

(Figs. 91–98)

Specific characters:

Body broadly ovate, elliptical with rounded posterior end; oral sucker smaller than ventral sucker; prepharynx very short; caeca lateral, unbranched, extending from pharynx to subcaudal region; testes and ovary branched, cirrus sac sinuous.

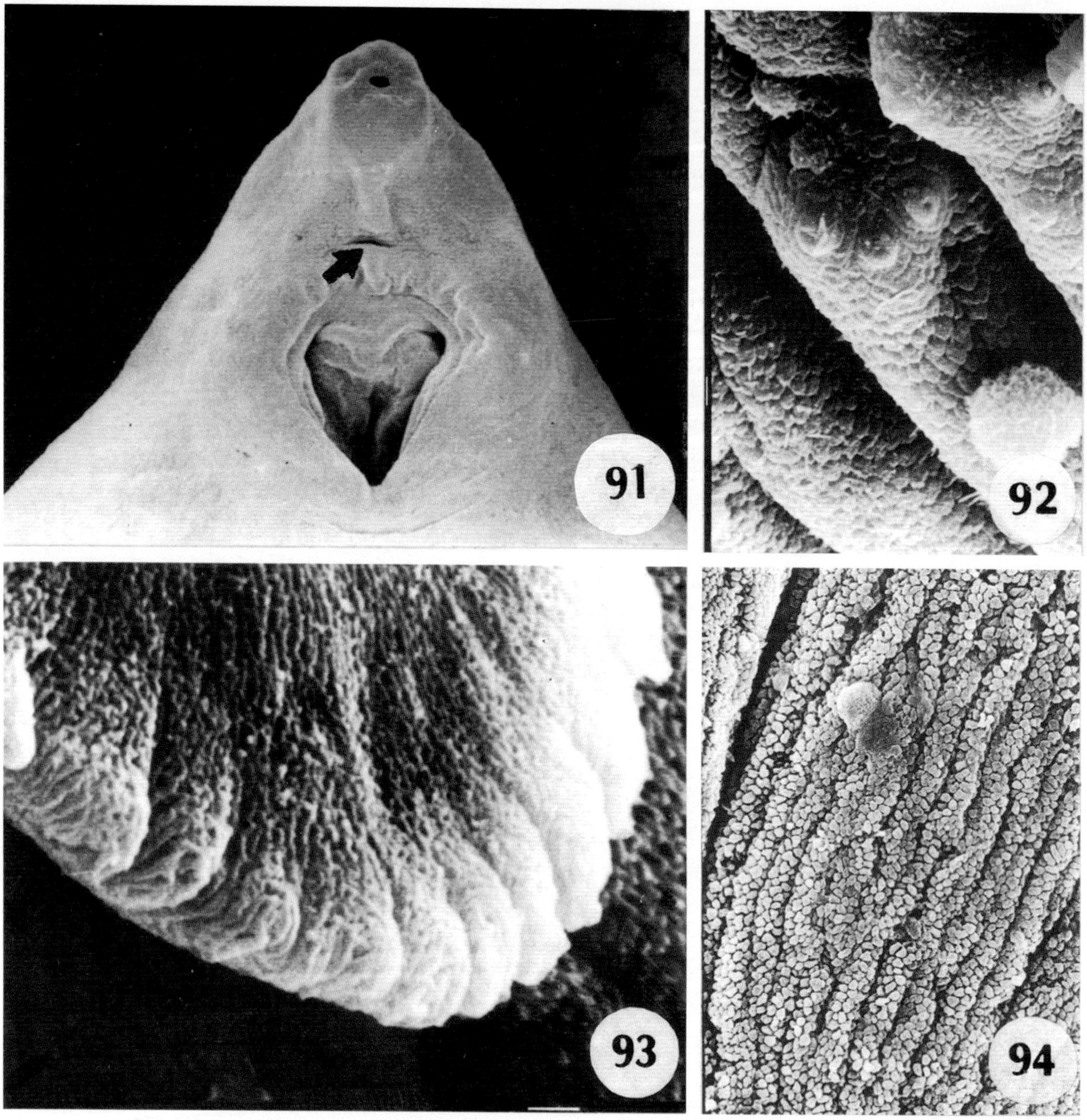

Figs. 91–94. *Fasciolopsis buski.*
91: Anterior region of body, showing oral sucker, ventral sucker and genital pore opening (arrow). × 44
92: Inner wall of acetabulum, showing clustered domed papillae. × 5400
93: One ventral scale enlarged. × 8000
94: Enlarged view of general body surface, showing fine tuberculation of body. × 2000

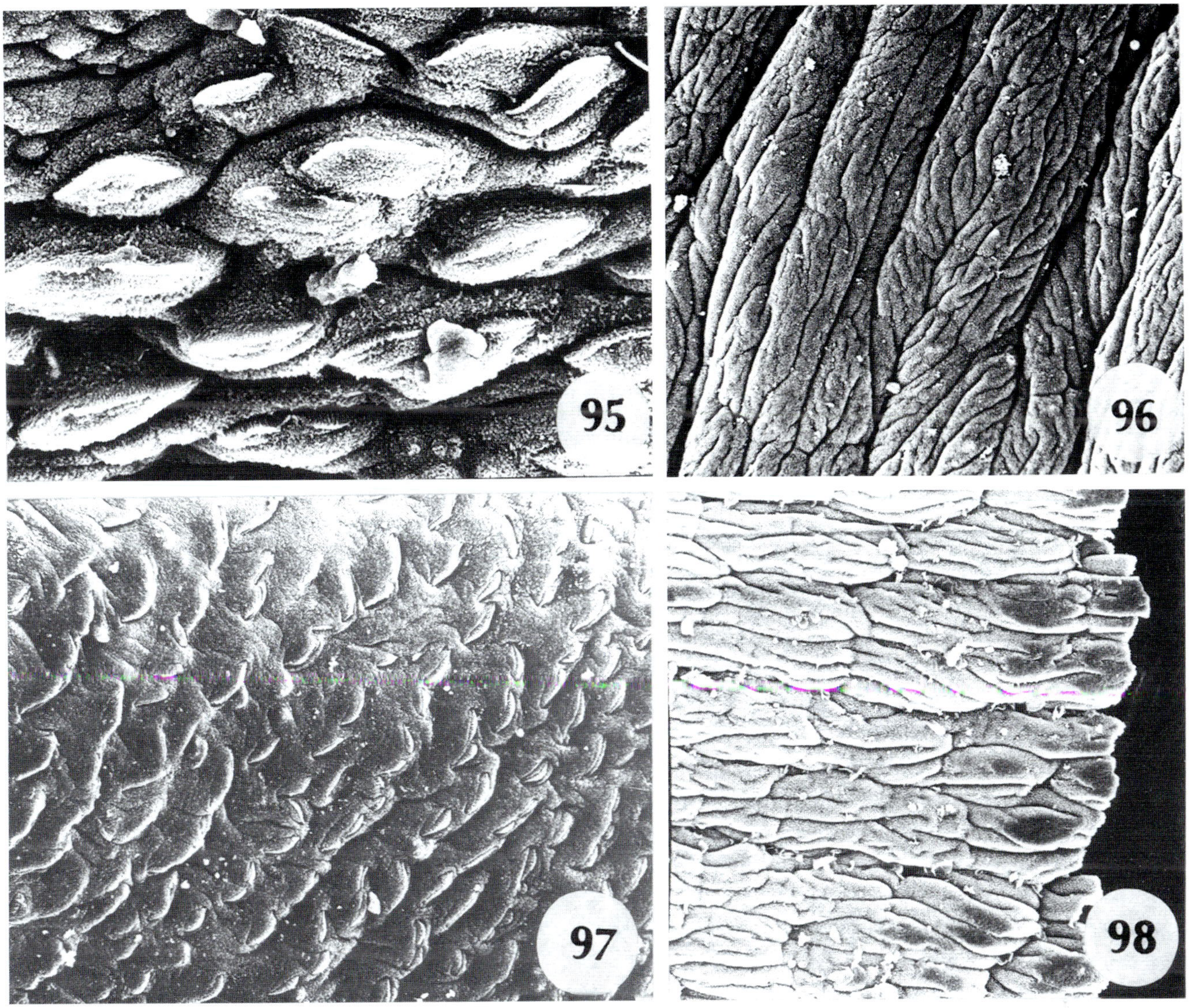

Figs. 95–98. *Fasciolopsis buski.*
95: Tegument of the region between suckers, showing elliptical papillae. × 1500
96: Dorsal surface of body. × 400
97: The region posterior to ventral sucker, showing scale-like structures. × 660
98: Lateral edge of body, dorsal surface. × 360

Genus : *Eurytrema* Looss, 1907
Host : *Bos indicus*, *Bubalus bubalis*, *Ovis aries*, *Capra hircus*
Habitat : Bile duct
Species : *Eurytrema pancreaticum* (Janson, 1889) Looss, 1907

(Figs. 99–102)

Specific characters:

Flattened body with ruffled margins and conical caudal appendage, oral sucker larger than ventral sucker, caeca narrow, reaching to posterior part of body; testes irregular in shape, posterolateral to ventral sucker, cirrus sac elongated; ovary subterminal, vitellaria small finger-like follicles in lateral fields; genital pore postbifurcal.

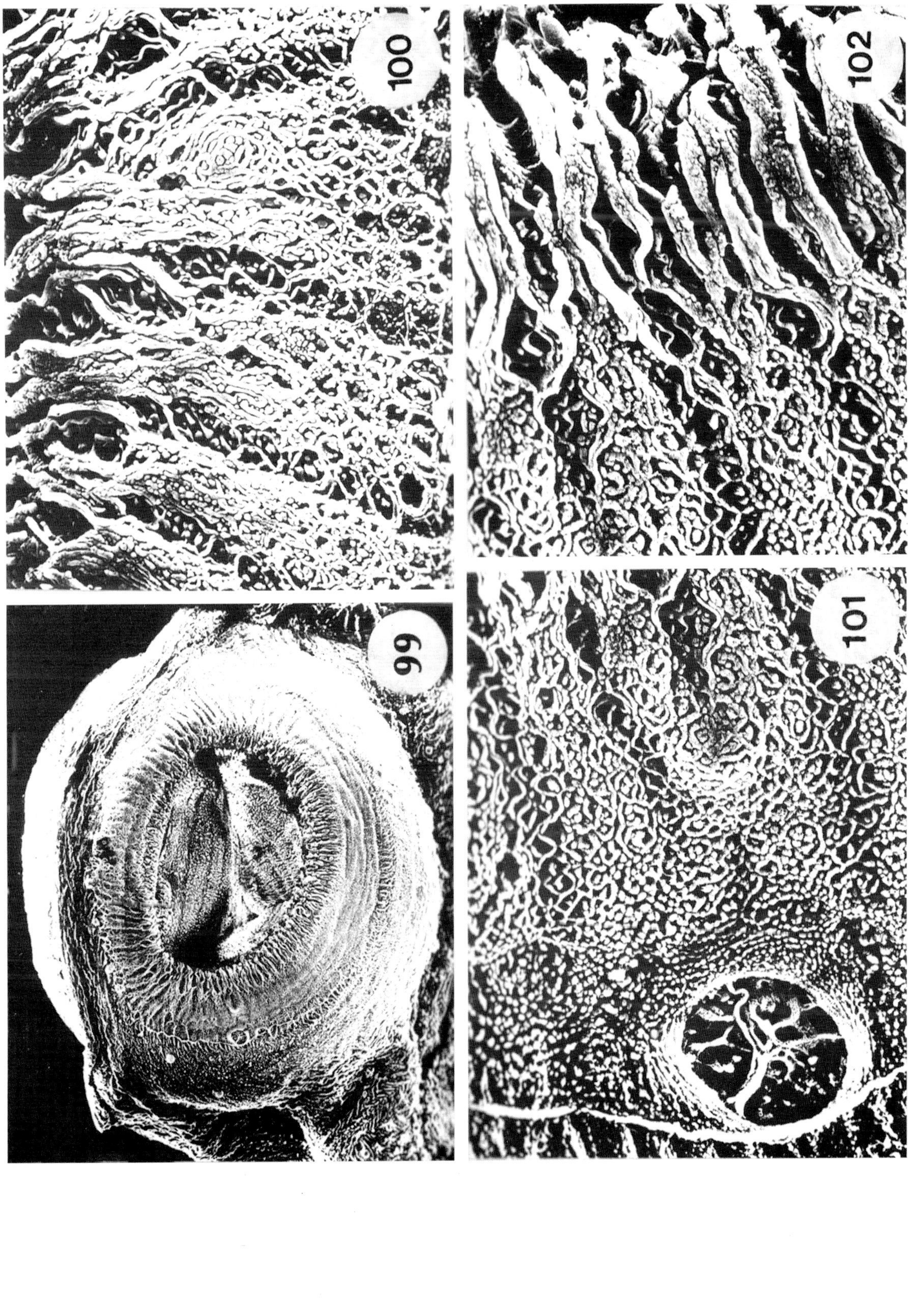

Figs. 99–102. *Eurytrema pancreaticum.*
99: Oral sucker. × 100
100: Rim of oral sucker. Note the conspicuous transverse foldings of tegument. × 860
101: Distal region of oral rim, showing intricate network of tegumental folds just behind the radial tegumental foldings. × 1000
102: A closer view of the proximal part, showing radially extending tegumental foldings. × 1200

Genus : *Opisthorchis* Blanchard, 1895
Host : *Sus scrofa domestica, Bos indicus* (accidental)
Habitat : Bile duct
Species : *Opisthorchis noverca* Braun, 1902

(Figs. 103–105 and 107 pig origin; 106, cattle origin)

Specific characters:

Flattened and elongated body, oral sucker larger than ventral sucker; oesophagus short, caeca more or less straight reaching up to posterior end of body; testes rounded or lobate in posterior third of body; irregularly lobed ovary; vitellaria in lateral fields with eight follicle groups; excretory vesicle 'Y'-shaped, stem passing between testes.

Figs. 103–107. *Opisthorchis noverca.*
103: Whole worm, ventral view. × 20
104: Anterior region of worm, showing heavy spination of body surface. × 180
105: A closer view of tegumental spines. × 2000
106: Shovel-shaped tegumental spines. The difference in the shape of spines in flukes of cattle origin may be due to difference in the habitat. × 2000
107: Surface topography in the region of ventral sucker. × 540

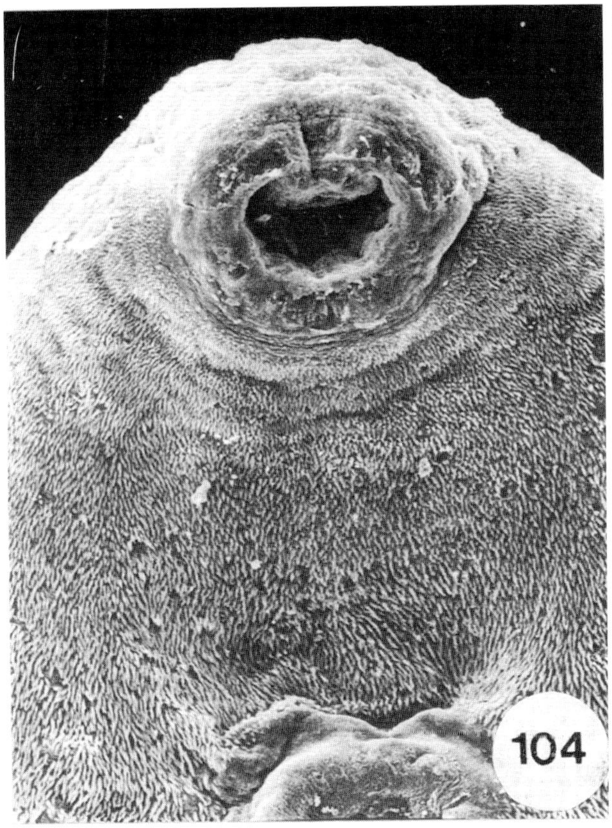
104

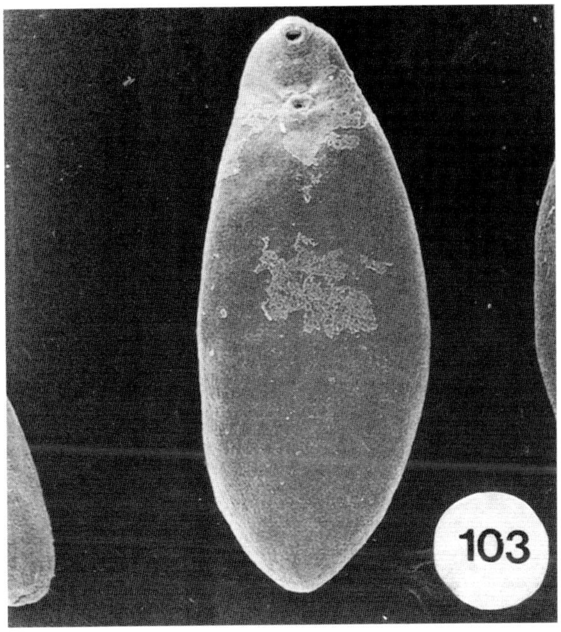
103

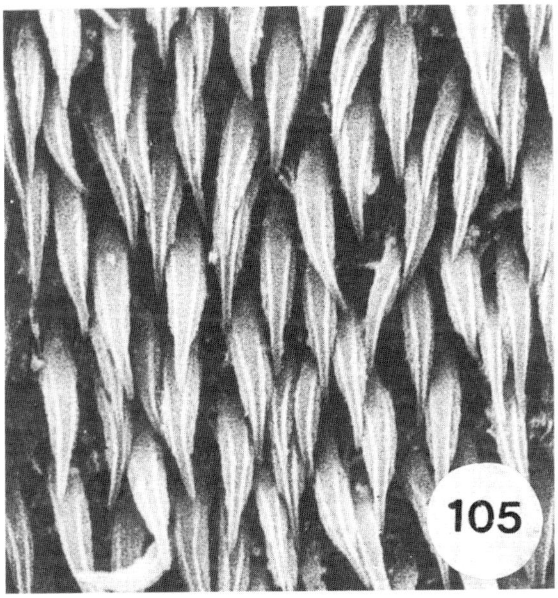
105

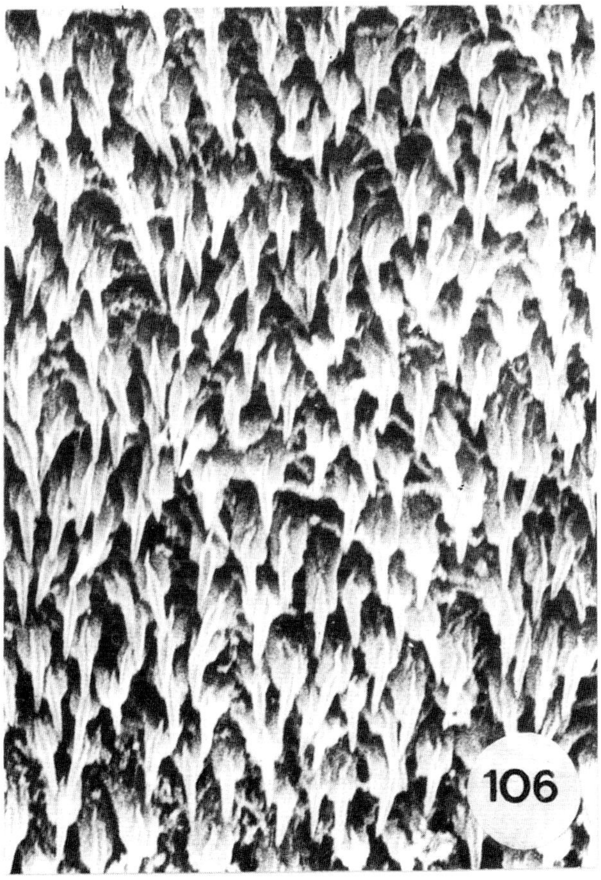
106

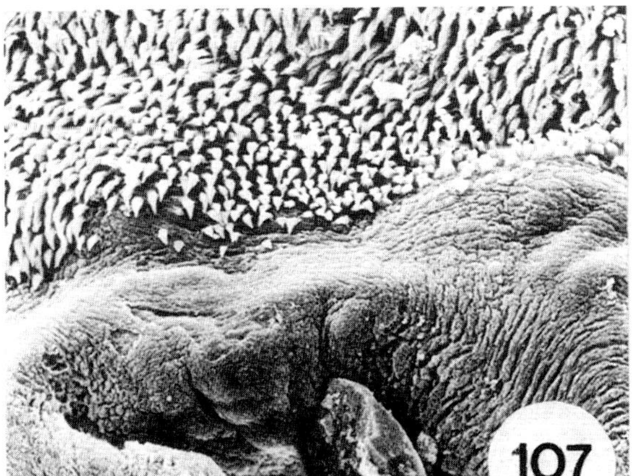
107

Genus : *Artyfechinostomum* Lane, 1915
Host : *Sus scrofa domestica*
Habitat : Intestine
Species : *Artyfechinostomum sufrartyfex* (Leiper, 1911) Railliet, 1925
[Syn. *Euparyphium malayanum* Leiper, 1911
Artyfechinostomum sufrartyfex, Lane, 1915
Testifrondosa cristata Bhalerao, 1924
Paryphostomum mehrai of Jain, 1957
Neoartyfechinostomum shubhrai Agrawal, 1963
Echinostoma rehmani Rao et Niphadper, 1963]

(Figs. 108–115)

Specific characters:

Conical body having 39 collar spines, five spines in each corner group; ventral sucker postbifurcal; caeca wavy, reaching up to posterior end; testes branched, post equatorial; ovary rounded or spherical; uterus intercaecal, transversely coiled between anterior testis and acetabulum; genital opening preacetabular, postbifurcal.

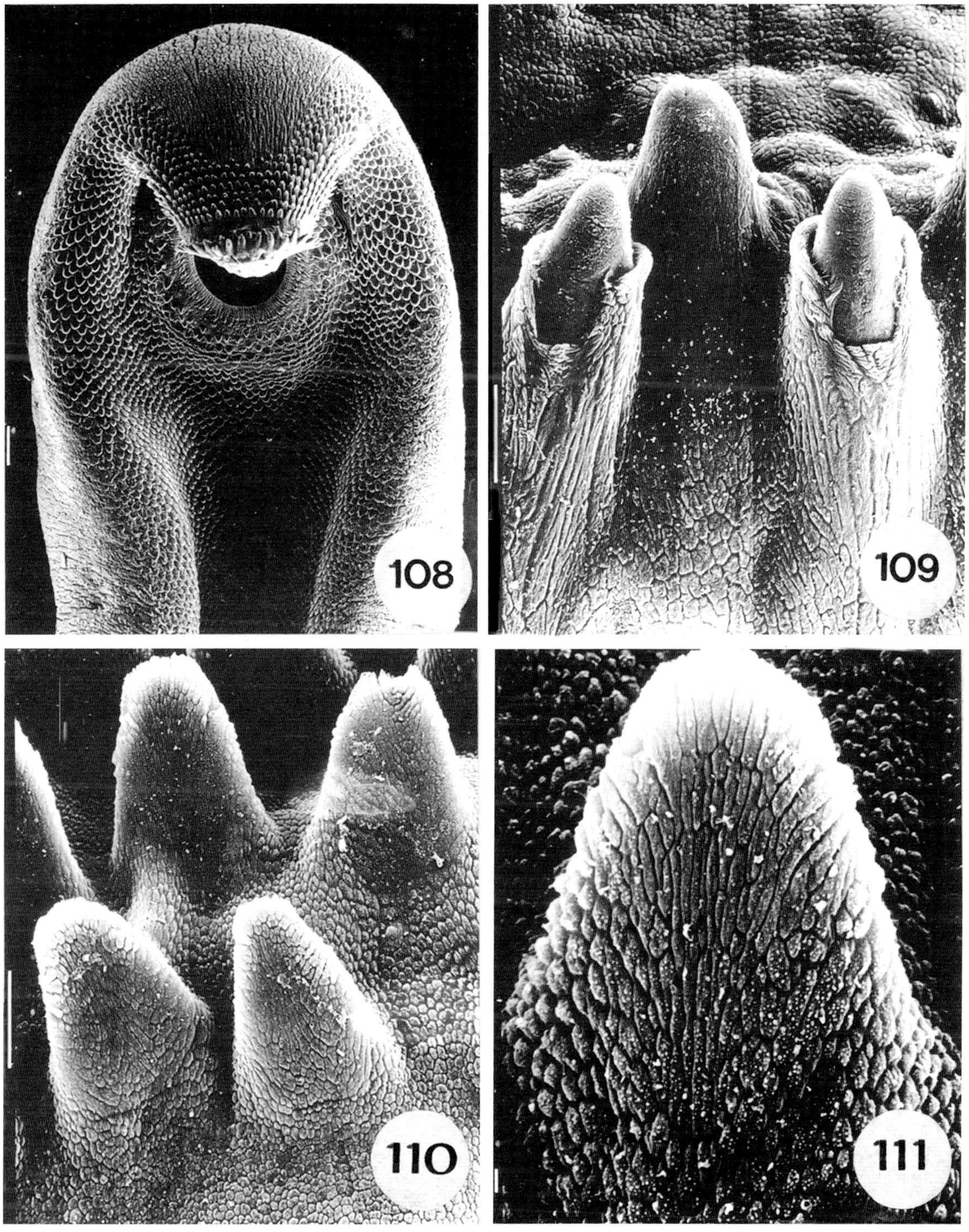

Figs. 108–111. *Artyfechinostomum sufrartyfex.*
108: Anterior region of body, ventral view. × 66
109: Collar spines, in a closer view, revealing the socketed and non-socketed types. × 1600
110: Spines on dorsal surface. × 1600
111: A single dorsal spine in an enlarged view, revealing mosaic corrugation of its surface. × 4000

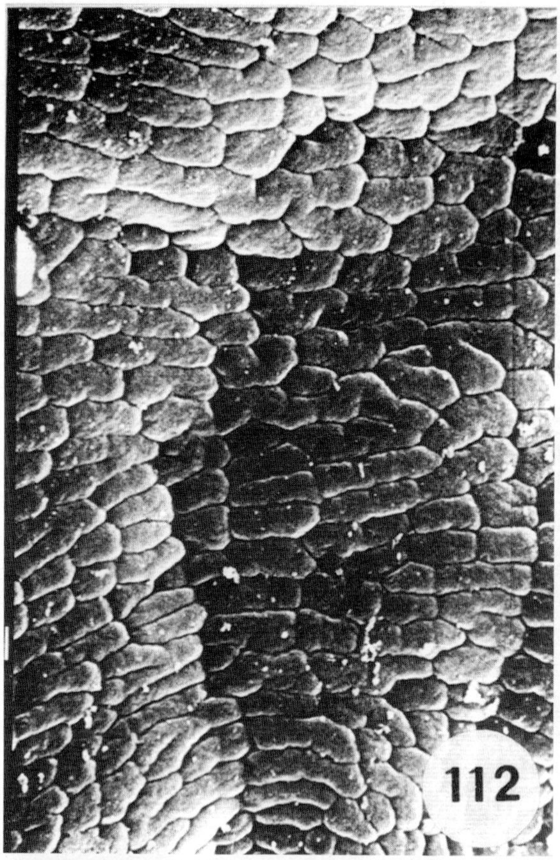
112

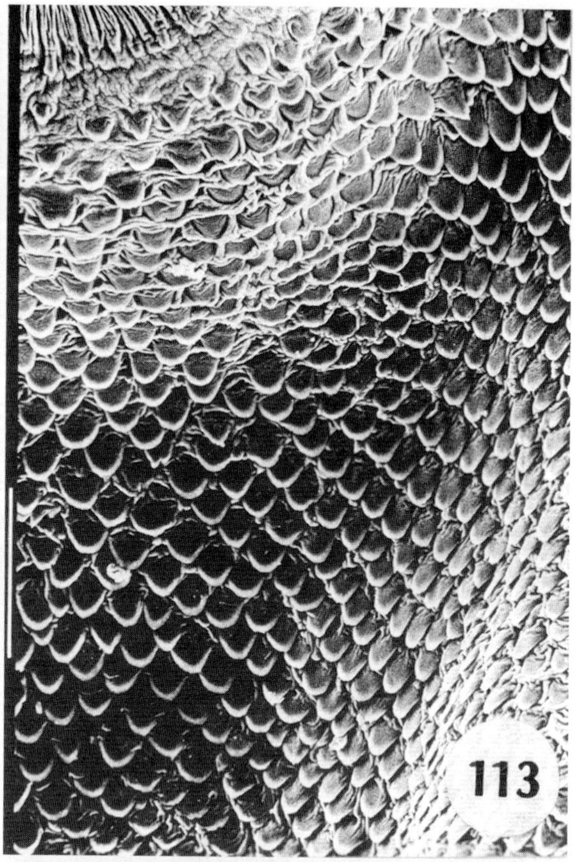
113

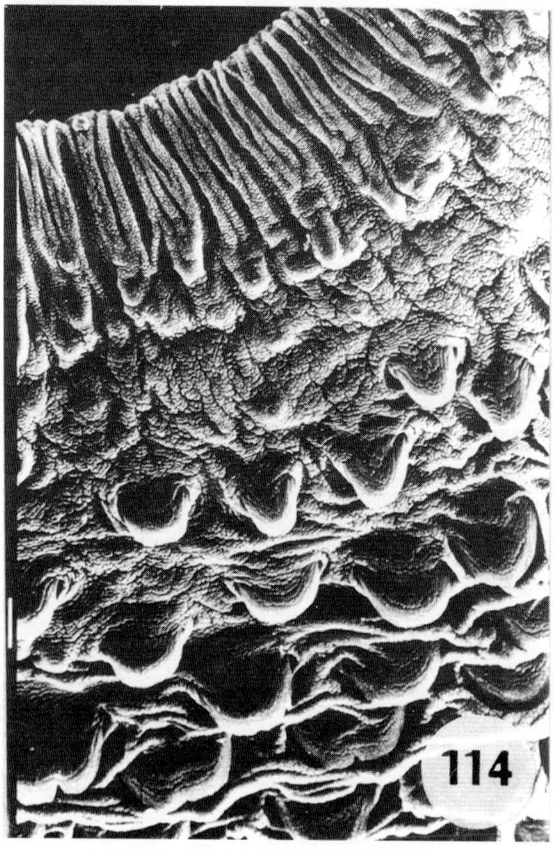
114

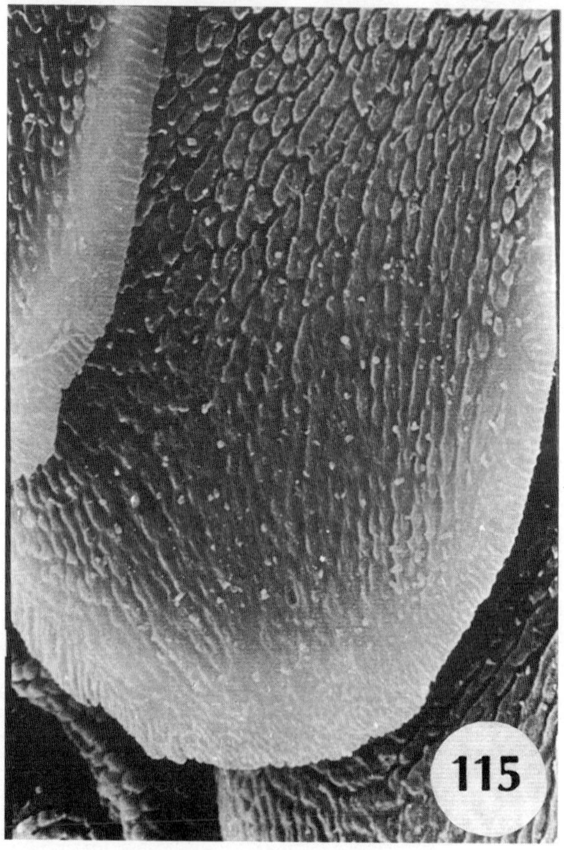
115

Genus : *Echinostoma* Rudolphi, 1809
Host : *Gallus gallus domestica*
Habitat : Intestine
Species : *Echinostoma revolutum* (Froelich, 1802) Looss, 1899

(Figs. 116–121)

Specific characters:

Body elongated, spined; collar spines 37 in number, 5 spines in each corner group; prepharynx distinct; genital pore preacetabular; testes tandem, postequatorial; cirrus sac relatively small, encroaching on anterior face of acetabulum; Mehlis' gland a little behind acetabulum; uterus intercaecal, transversely coiled between anterior testis and acetabulum.

Figs. 112–115. *Artyfechinostomum sufrartyfex.*
112: Dorsal surface, revealing the mosaic arrangement of plates. × 4800
113: Ventral surface, showing dense spination. × 240
114: A portion of ventral sucker and adjoining ventral surface. The rim is radially corrugated and is not smooth. × 720
115: A closer view of a single ventral spine. × 4000

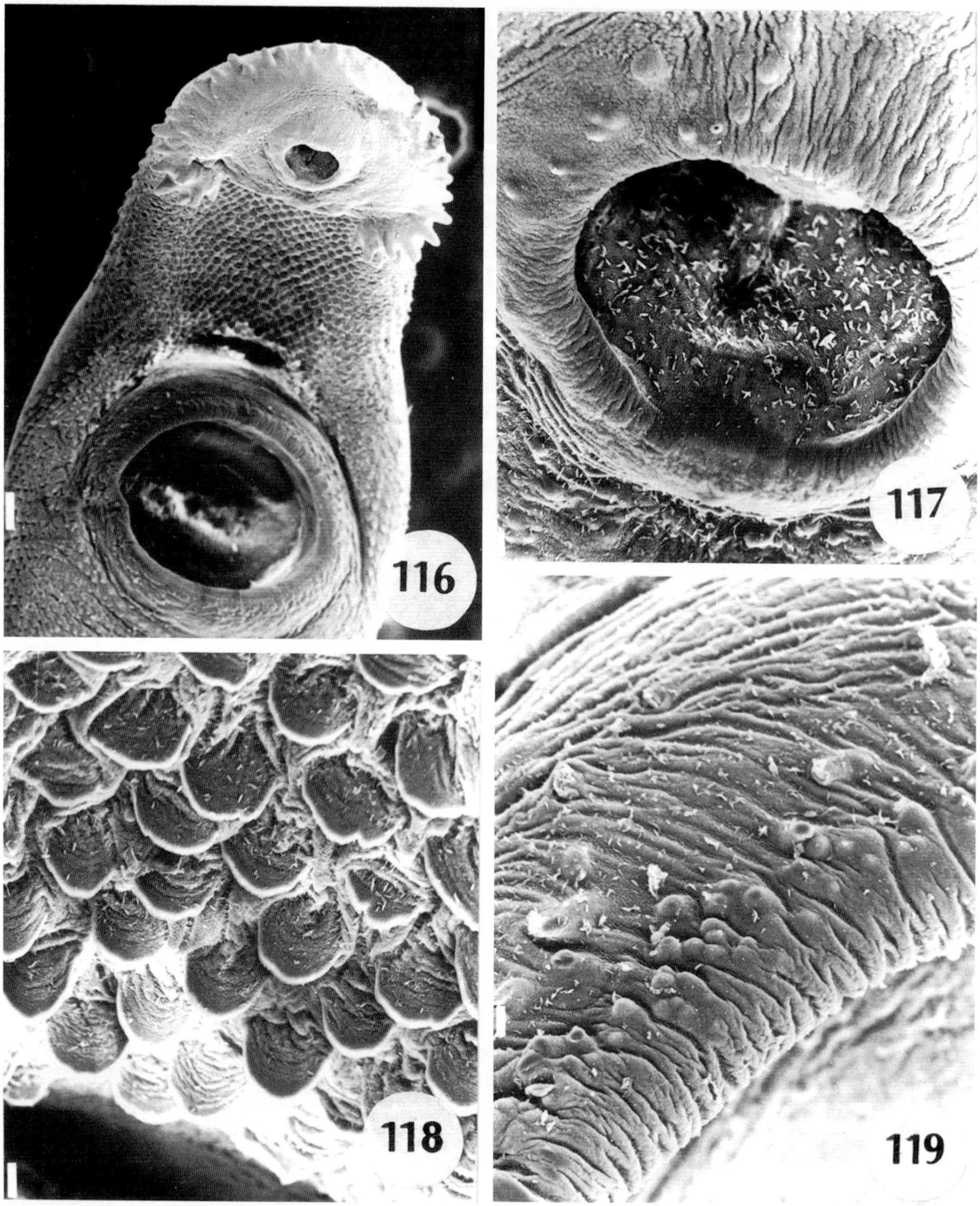

Figs. 116–119. *Echinostoma revolutum.*
116: Anterior part of body (ventral view), showing oral sucker, ventral sucker and collar spines. × 44
117: Oral sucker, ventral view. Sparsely distributed domed tuberculations are visible. × 440
118: Enlarged view of scale-like spines in the space between oral and ventral sucker. × 600
119: Rim of ventral sucker (enlarged view), showing radial foldings and dome-like papillae. × 540

Genus : *Catatropis* Odhner, 1905
Host : *Gallus gallus domestica*
Habitat : Caecum
Species : *Catatropis indicus* Srivastava, 1935

(Figs. 122–128)

Specific characters:

Elongated body; ventral surface concave; ventral glands in three rows, non-protrusible, continuous in median row; caeca provided with numerous minute diverticula; testes deeply lobed; cirrus sac median, flask shaped, with long neck; genital pore median, close behind oral sucker; irregularly lobed ovary; vitellaria from behind middle of body to a little beyond anterior end of testes.

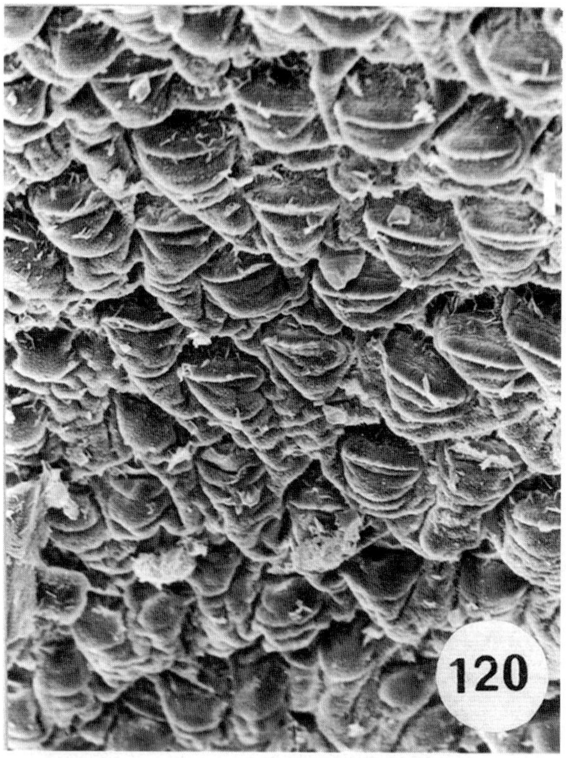

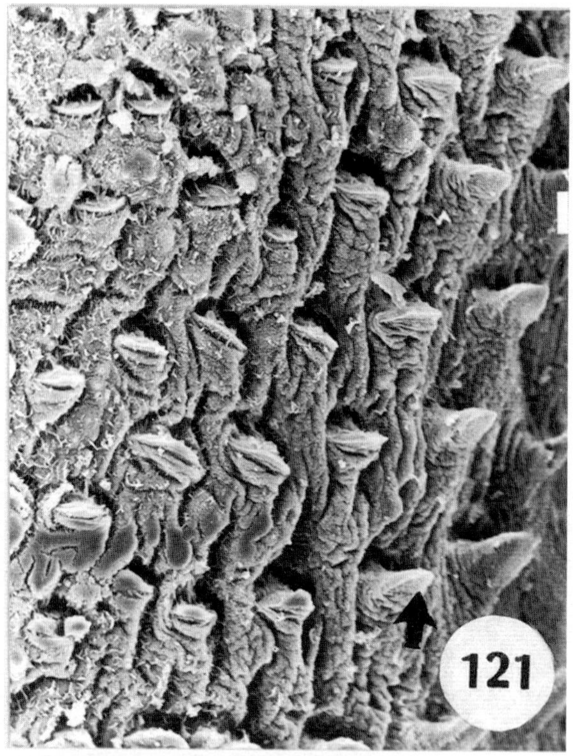

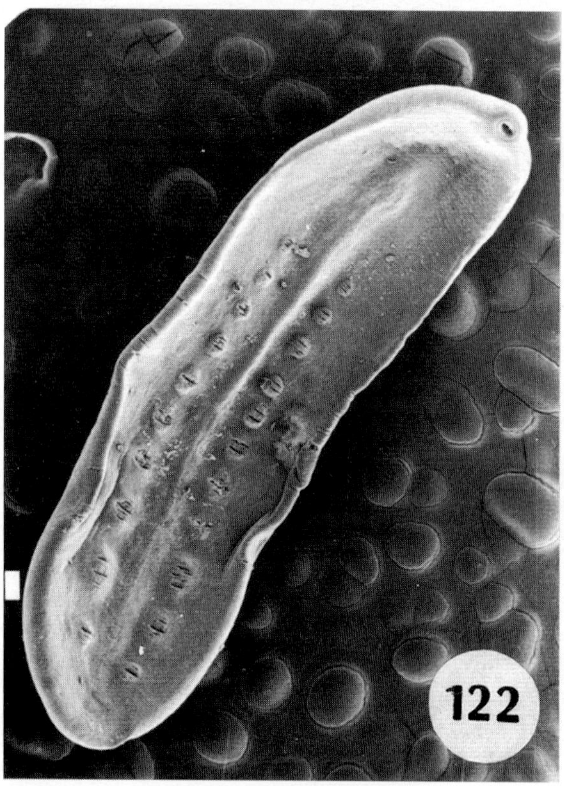

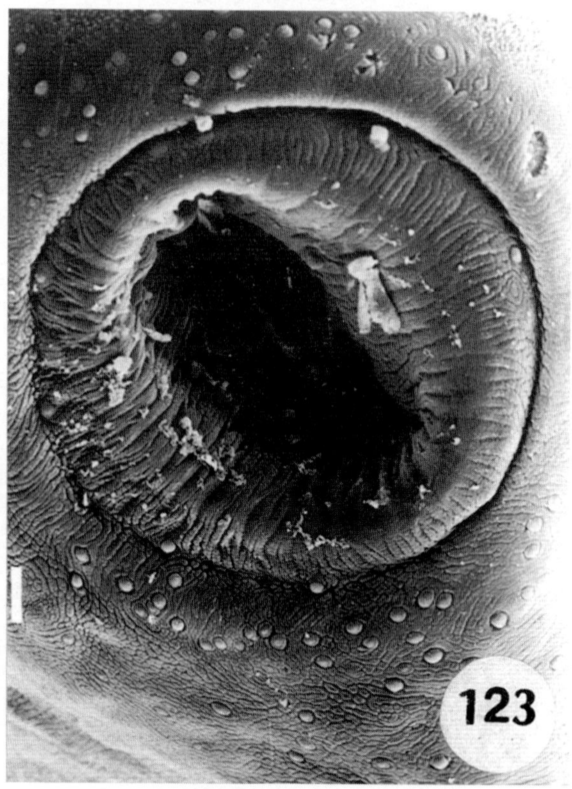

Figs. 120, 121. *Echinostoma revolutum.*
120: Ventral tegumentary scale-like structures in the region behind the ventral sucker. × 600
121: Peg-like spines in the ventrolateral field (arrow). × 600

Figs. 122, 123. *Catatropis indicus.*
122: Whole worm, ventral view showing arrangement of ventral glands on two sides of ventral ridge. × 44
123: Oral aperture in enlarged view, showing radial corrugations of the rim and rounded papillae surrounding the aperture. × 860

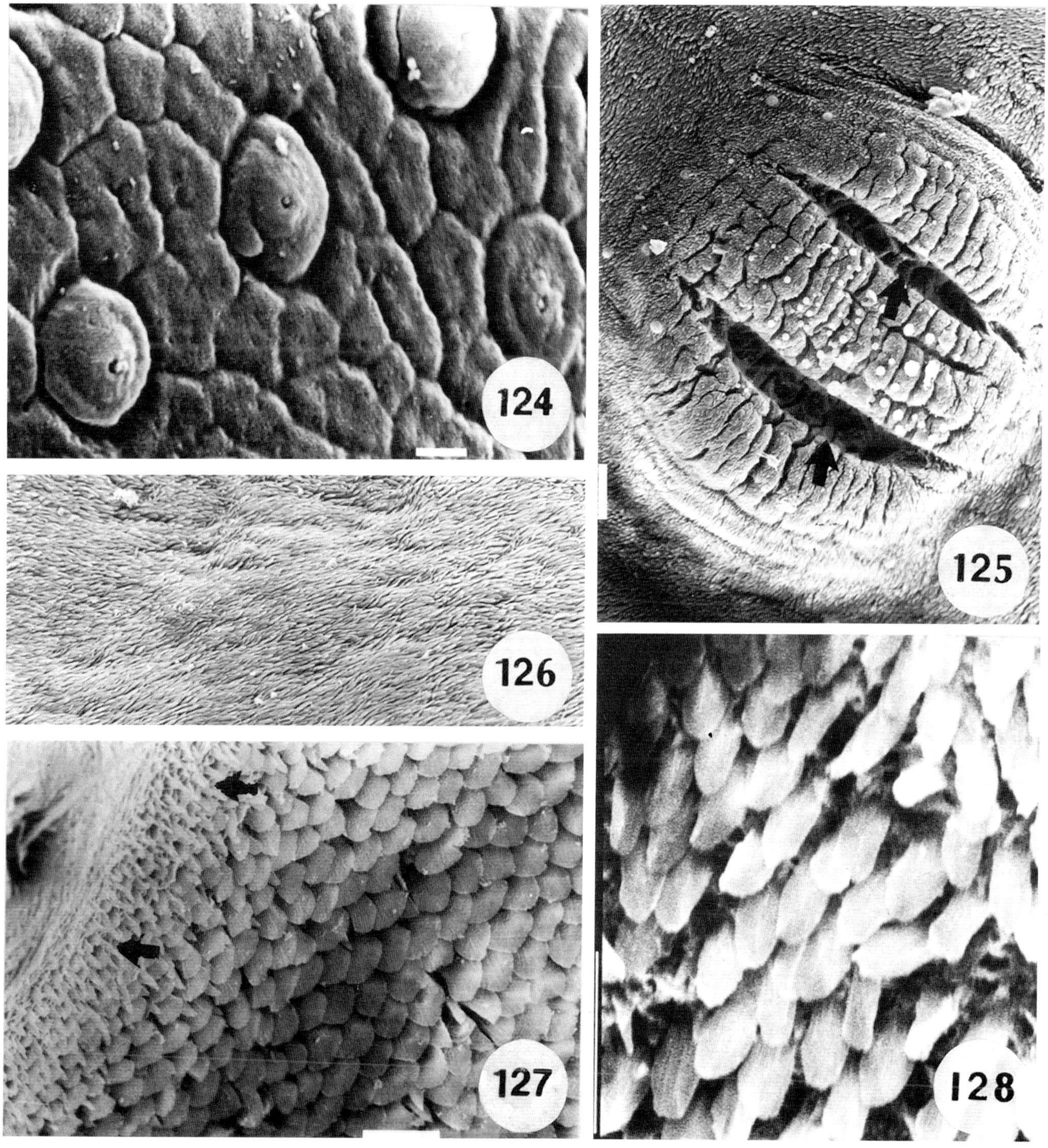

Figs. 124–128. *Catatropis indicus.*
124: Enlarged tegumental surface surrounding the oral aperture, showing smooth and ciliate papillae. × 10,000
125: One ventral gland, enlarged. Opening of the gland is prominent (arrows). × 1000
126: Ciliated body surface surrounding the ventral glands. × 1500
127: The portion behind the genital opening, showing dense spines (arrows) and scales. × 1500
128: Enlarged view of cilia with blunt tip. × 3200

Appendix

Types of Acetabulum (Fig. 129)

Calicophoron type (sensu Näsmark, 1937): dorsal exterior circular muscles (d.e.c.m.) and ventral exterior circular muscles (v.e.c.m.) not divided into two parts, dorsal and ventral halves of exterior circular musculature practically identical; radial muscle fibres moderately coarse, run individually.

Cotylophoron type (sensu Näsmark, 1937): similar to calicophoron type; however, differs from the latter in that both d.e.c.m. and v.e.c.m. are clearly separated from the interior acetabulum tissue by an obliquely running, longitudinally branched muscle band.

Explanatum type (sensu Näsmark, 1937): d.e.c.m. divided into two parts, d.e.c.m. 1 and d.e.c.m. 2; former very strongly developed; limit towards d.e.c.m. 2 very sharp and clear.

Gastrothylax type (sensu Näsmark, 1937): inner cavity of acetabulum basin shaped, bottom often forming a more or less level surface at right angles to the walls; d.e.c.m. and v.e.c.m. units displaying a very large number of units which exceeds that of units in dorsal interior circular muscles (d.i.c.m.) and ventral interior circular muscles (v.i.c.m.).

Homalogaster type (sensu Sey, 1984 with amendment by Jones, 1986): v.e.c.m. divided into two groups by obliquely running fibres; no distinct division of d.e.c.m.; interior series increasing in unit size away from sucker rim, then decreasing to smaller units internally; exterior series having a few irregular enlarged units near sucker rim; sucker shape in sagittal section characteristically asymmetrical, excavated anteriorly.

Paramphistomum type (sensu Näsmark, 1937): d.e.c.m. divided into two parts-d.e.c.m. 1 and d.e.c.m. 2; d.e.c.m. 1 strong, corresponding to entire v.e.c.m.

Pisum type (sensu Näsmark, 1937): d.e.c.m. divided into two parts; d.e.c.m. 2 slightly more developed (fewer units) than in paramphistomum type; an obliquely longitudinal muscle band limits d.e.c.m. 1 and v.e.c.m. from inner acetabulum tissue.

Stichorchis type (sensu Näsmark, 1937): units in d.e. and v.e. circular series very close to each other at the margin of acetabulum; i.c.m. series spread over a large part of inner acetabulum periphery, numerous thick lymphatic ramifications present in between radial muscle fibres of acetabular tissue.

Streptocoelium type (sensu Näsmark, 1937): d.e.c.m. and v.e.c.m. relatively slightly developed, units almost equal in size, perhaps somewhat smaller at beginning and end of series; d.i.c.m. and v.i.c.m. units more in number than exterior ones, also more strongly developed. Interior circular series forming an even arc-shaped curve, having smallest units at beginning and end of series.

Watsonius type (sensu Näsmark, 1937): c.m. units are more strongly developed in exterior series, somewhat smaller in middle part of sucker but approximately uniform in size.

Types of Pharynx (Fig. 130)

Calicophoron type (sensu Dinnik, 1964): primary pharyngeal sacs absent, lip sphincter lacking; internal surface lined by small dome-shaped papillae; middle circular muscle layer may or may not be present.

Dicranocoelium type (sensu Näsmark, 1937): pharyngeal sacs absent, middle circular muscle layer lacking; lip sphincter present.

Explanatum type (sensu Näsmark, 1937): primary pharyngeal sacs absent, middle circular muscle layer present; exterior circular muscle layer present, but developed only in anterior part of pharynx; both anterior and posterior pharyngeal sphincters present; units of interior circular muscle layer strongly developed.

Homalogaster type (sensu Sey, 1984): pharyngeal bulb, secondary pharyngeal sacs present; middle circular layer moderately developed; anterior muscle units biggest, loosely packed without forming an anterior sphincter; inner circular layer poorly developed; big papillae present around mouth opening.

Pisum type (sensu Näsmark, 1937): pharynx without pharyngeal bulb; primary pharyngeal sacs absent; middle circular muscle layer present; units of interior circular muscle layers very strongly developed; exterior circular muscle layer relatively poorly developed.

Watsonius type (sensu Näsmark, 1937): pharyngeal bulb, secondary pharyngeal sacs present; anterior pharyngeal sphincter absent; middle circular layer with very strongly developed units.

Types of Terminal Genitalium (Fig. 131)

Calicophoron type (sensu Näsmark, 1937): genital atrium lying exposed at top of a "ventral papilla" situated in centre of a large flat ventral atrium; genital sphincter, sphincter papillae present; latter closely packed; radial musculature of ventral atrium and genital atrium well-developed.

Cotylophoron type (sensu Näsmark, 1937): genital atrium divided to form so-called genital sucker, having clear delimiting membrane against tissues of body.

Dawesi type (sensu Eduardo, 1985): presence of round to oval genital sphincter, sphincter papilla absent.

Elongatus type (sensu Sey, 1983): genital papillae, median papillae provided with genital sphincter and ventral sphincter; tegumental papillae present only in median papilla.

Epiclitum type (sensu Näsmark, 1937): shallow genital atrium; prominent genital papilla; radial musculature of genital atrium distinct, well-developed; circular musculature entirely absent; wall of terminal genitalium semi-circular in outline, giving false impression of sucker; genital sphincter, sphincter papillae absent.

Explanatum type (sensu Näsmark, 1937): genital papilla of varied appearance in different stages of extension; genital sphincter absent; sphincter papillae present, of varied development, from being indistinct to very distinct; radial musculature of genital atrium well-developed.

Gracile type (sensu Näsmark, 1937): circular, radial musculature absent; wall of genital atrium strongly and uniformly developed, with a delimiting membrane against body tissue; genital sphincter, sphincter papillae absent.

Homalogaster type (sensu Sey, 1984): genital papilla large with swollen tip, genital fold very much conspicuous; genital sphincter absent; well-developed circular, longitudinal and dorsoventral muscle fibres present beneath area surrounding pore, their arrangement continuing uninterrupted to base of genital papilla.

Ichikawai type (sensu Näsmark, 1937): genital sphincter absent; genital papilla very thick, clumsy; sphincter papillae well-developed.

Microbothrium type (sensu Näsmark, 1937): genital sphincter considerable in size, well-delimited from surrounding tissue; sphincter papillae fairly strongly developed.

Orthocoelium type (sensu Eduardo,1985): large terminal genitalium; thick genital papilla, well-developed genital sphincter, sphincter papilla present.

Papillogenitalis type (sensu Eduardo, 1980): genital atrium provided with tegumental papillae on its wall; weakly developed genital sphincter, well-developed sphincter papilla present.

Parvipapillatum type (sensu Eduardo, 1985): genital sphincter, sphincter papilla absent; small tegumental papillae present on wall of genital fold.

Scoliocoelium type (sensu Näsmark, 1937): genital sphincter strongly developed; sphincter papilla also developed; slightly developed radial musculature; ventral atrium lacking.

Streptocoelium type (sensu Näsmark, 1937): genital papilla thick, clumsy; strong belt of muscle fibres of sphincter papillae present; units more strongly developed; radial musculature of genital atrium difficult to observe; sphincter papilla extensive, connected to well developed genital sphincter.

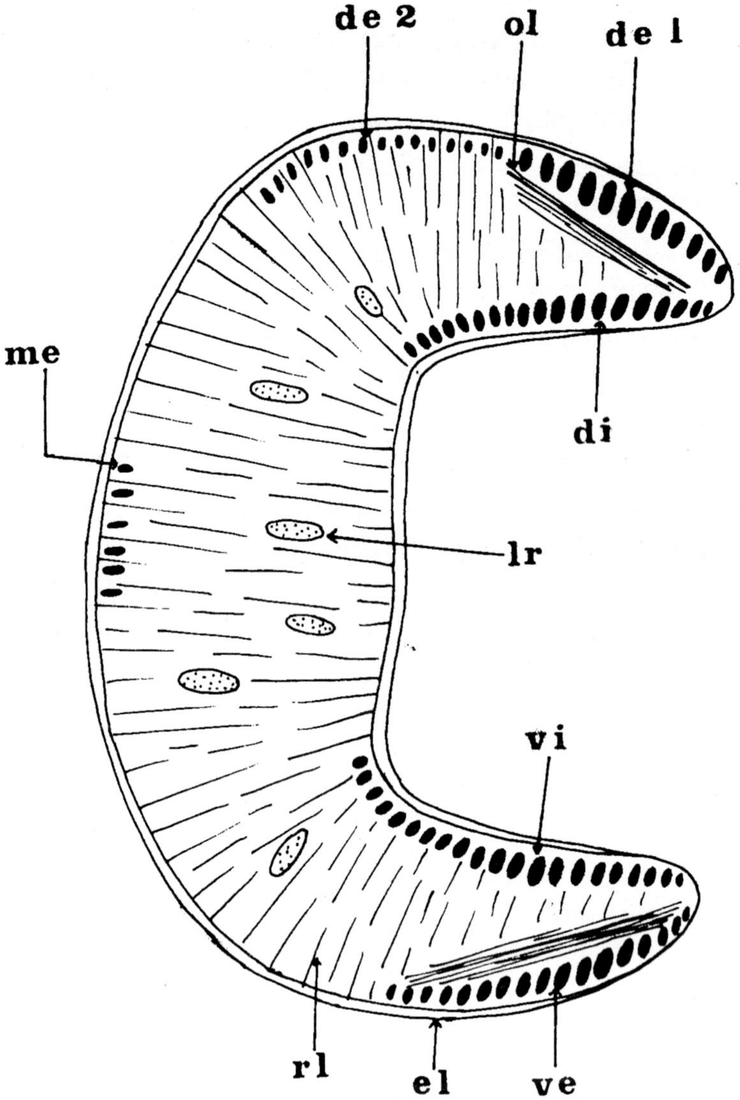

Fig. 129. Sagittal section of acetabulum (generalised) in amphistomes (de 1, dorsal exterior group1 muscles; de 2, dorsal exterior group 2 muscles; di, dorsal interior muscles; el, external lateral muscles; lr, longitudinal radial muscles; me, median exterior circular muscles; ol, oblique lateral muscles; rl, radial muscles; ve, ventral exterior muscles; vi, ventral interior muscles).

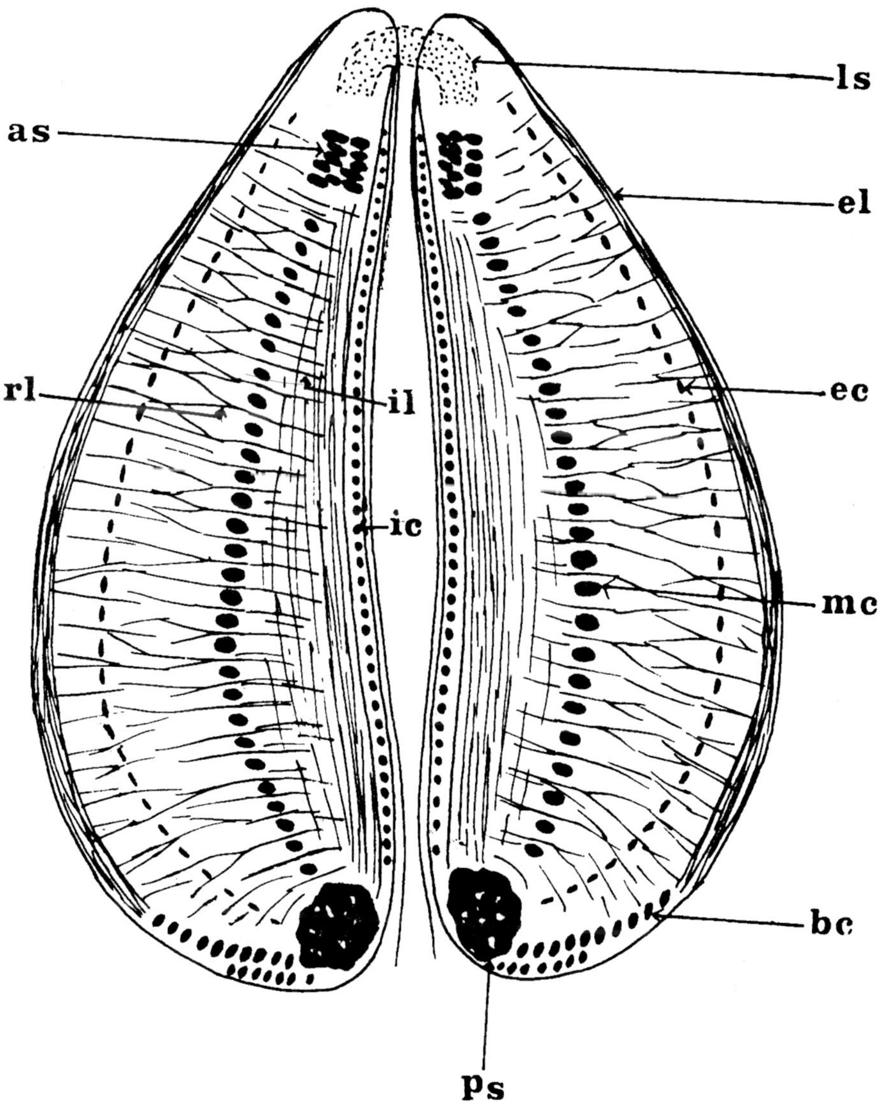

Fig. 130. Sagittal section of pharynx (generalised) in amphistomes (as, anterior sphincter; bc, basal circular muscles; ec, external circular muscles; el, external longitudinal muscles; ic, inner circular muscles; il, inner longitudinal muscles; mc, middle circular muscles; ps, posterior sphincter; rl, radial muscles).

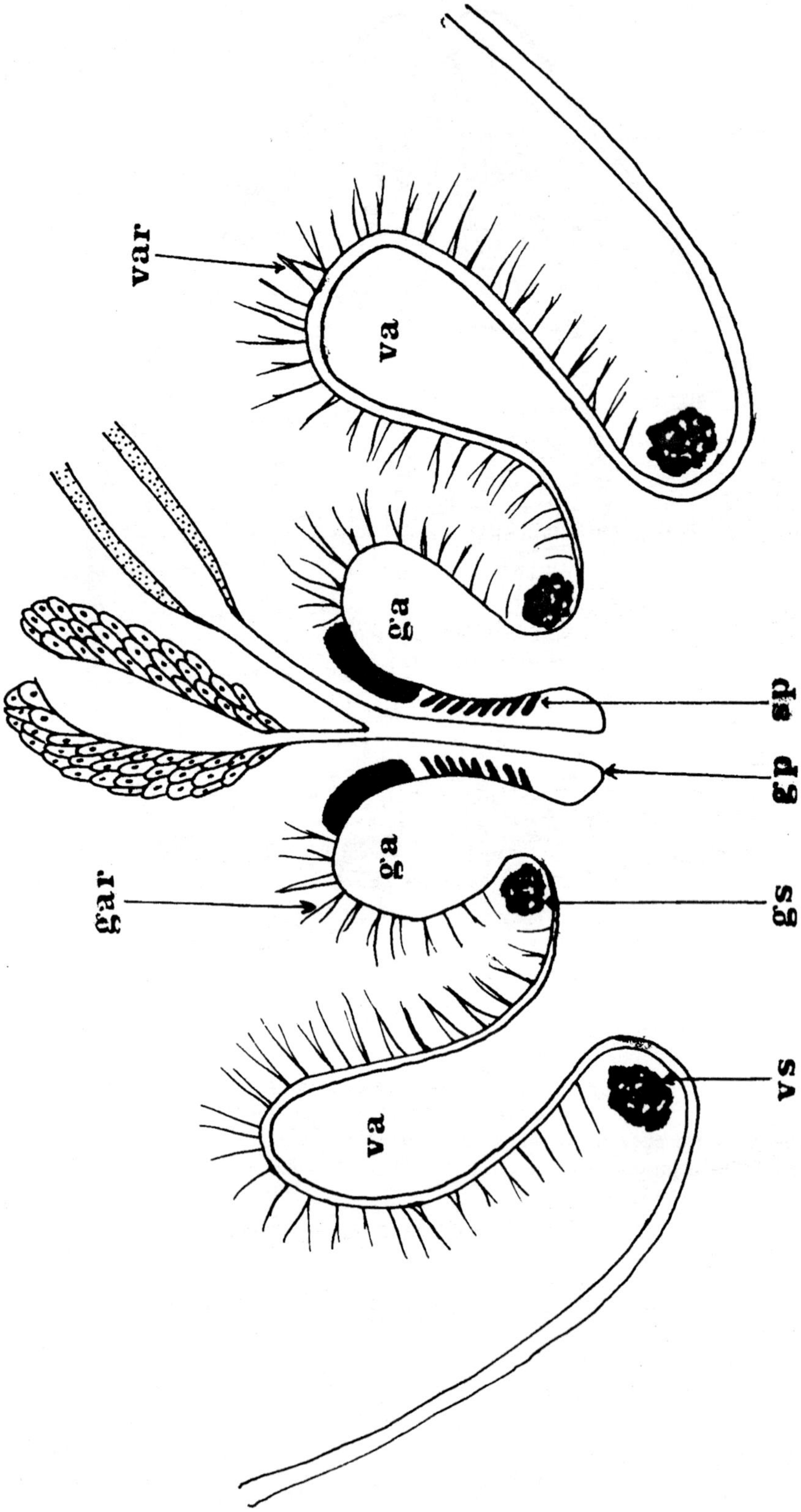

Fig. 131. Sagittal section of genitalium (generalised) in amphistomes (ga, genital atrium; gar, genital atrial radial muscles; gs, genital sphincter; gp, genital papilla; sp, sphincter papillae; va, ventral atrium; var, ventral atrial radial muscles; vs, ventral sphincter).

Plate I: Spectrum of digenetic trematodes: whole mounts (photomicrographs)

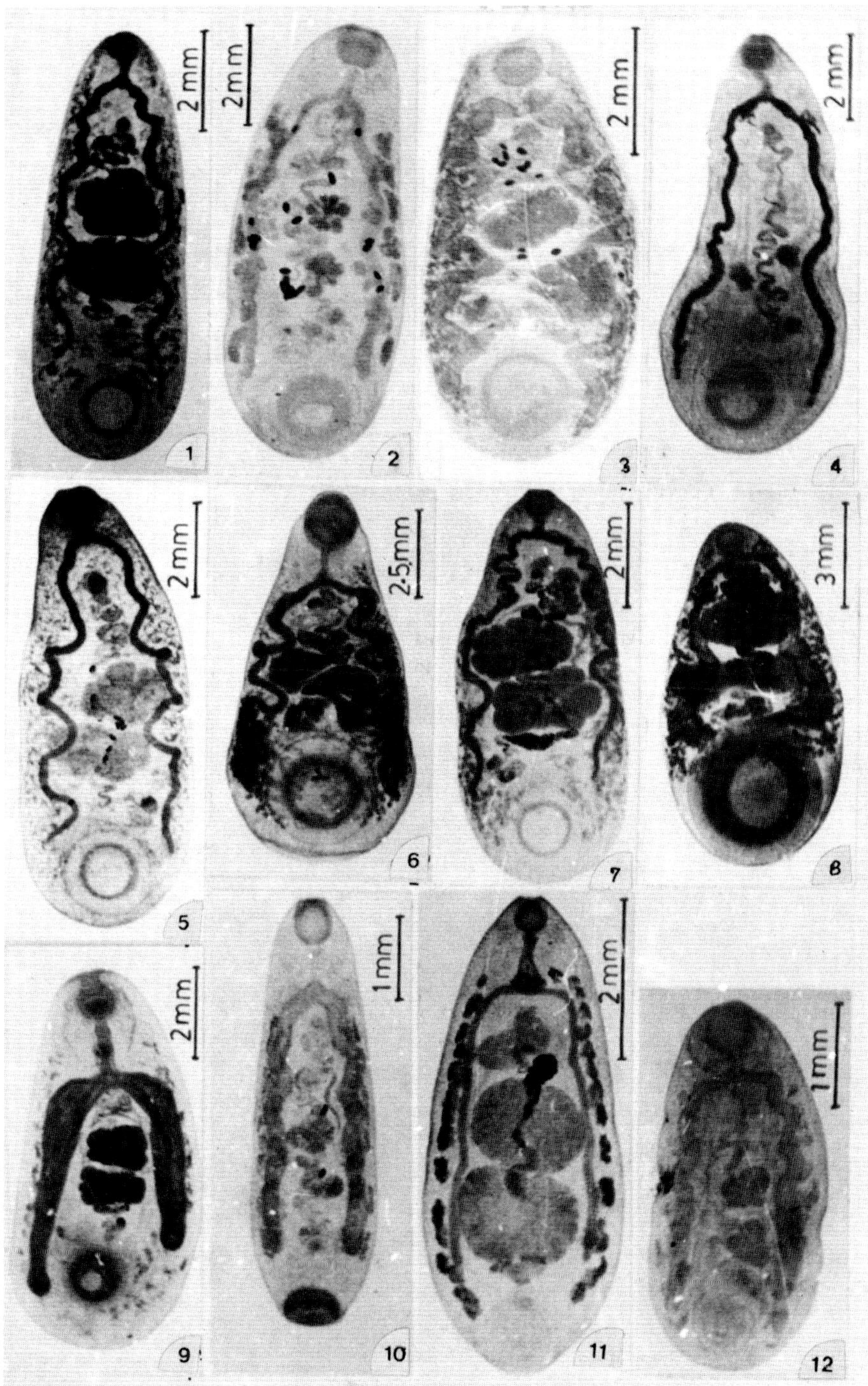

Fig. 1: *Paramphistomum epiclitum;* Fig. 2: *P. ichikawai;* Fig. 3: *P. gracile;* Fig. 4: *Calicophoron calicophorum;* Fig. 5: *C. papillosum;* Fig. 6: *C. shillongensis*; Fig. 7: *Cotylophoron cotylophorum*; Fig. 8: *Explanatum explanatum*; Fig. 9: *Orthocoelium orthocoelium*; Fig. 10: *O. dicranocoelium*; Fig. 11: *O. dawesi*; Fig. 12: *O. scoliocoelium*

Plate II: Spectrum of digenetic trematodes: whole mounts (photomicrographs)

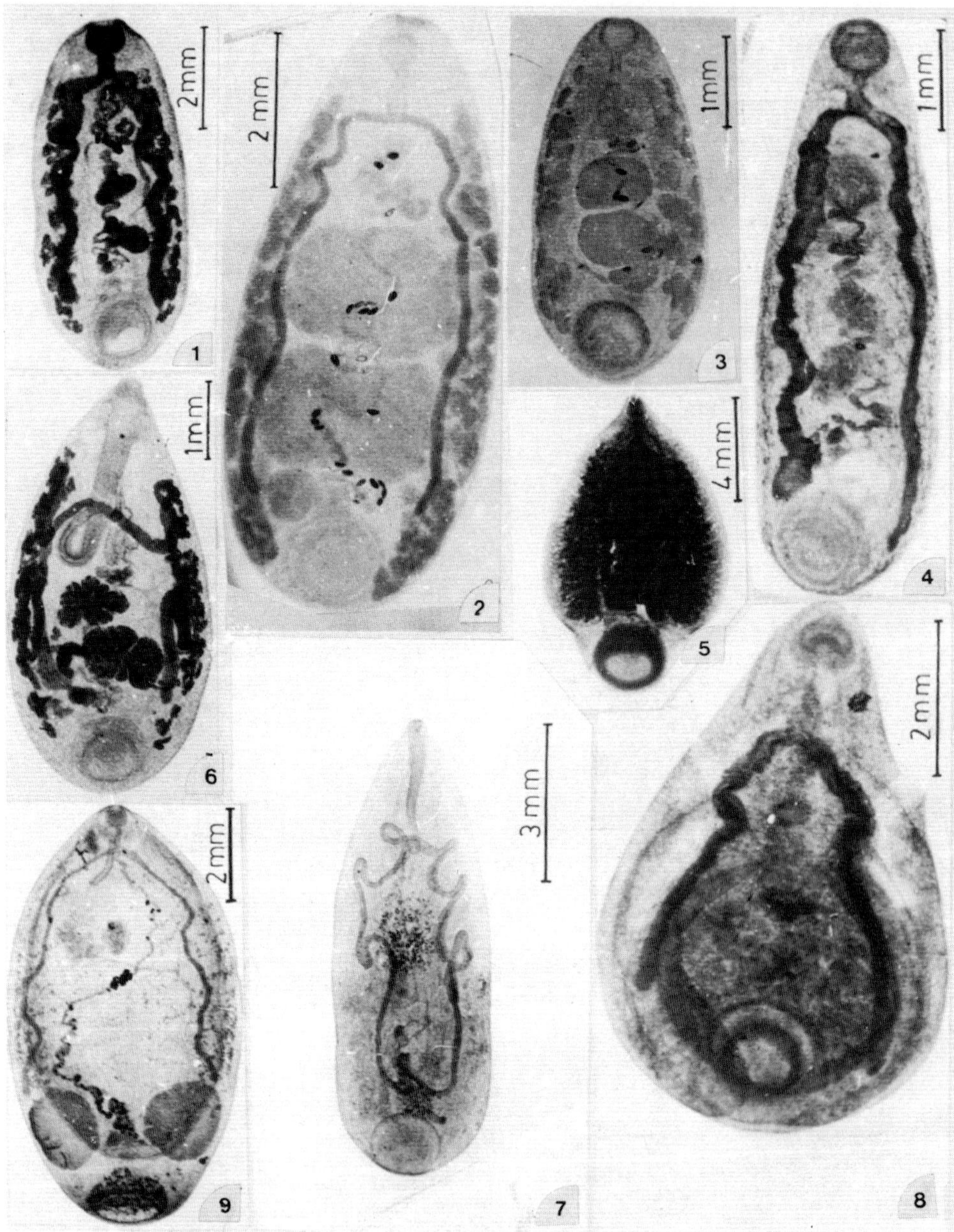

Fig. 1: *Orthocoelium streptocoelium*; Fig. 2: *O. parvipapillatum;* Fig. 3: *O. dinniki;* Fig. 4: *Leiperocotyle meghalayensis*; Fig. 5: *Homalogaster paloniae*; Fig. 6: *Olveria indica*; Fig. 7: *O. bosi;* Fig. 8: *Gastrodiscoides hominis*; Fig. 9: *Gastrothylax crumenifer*

Plate III: Spectrum of digenetic trematodes: whole mounts (photomicrographs)

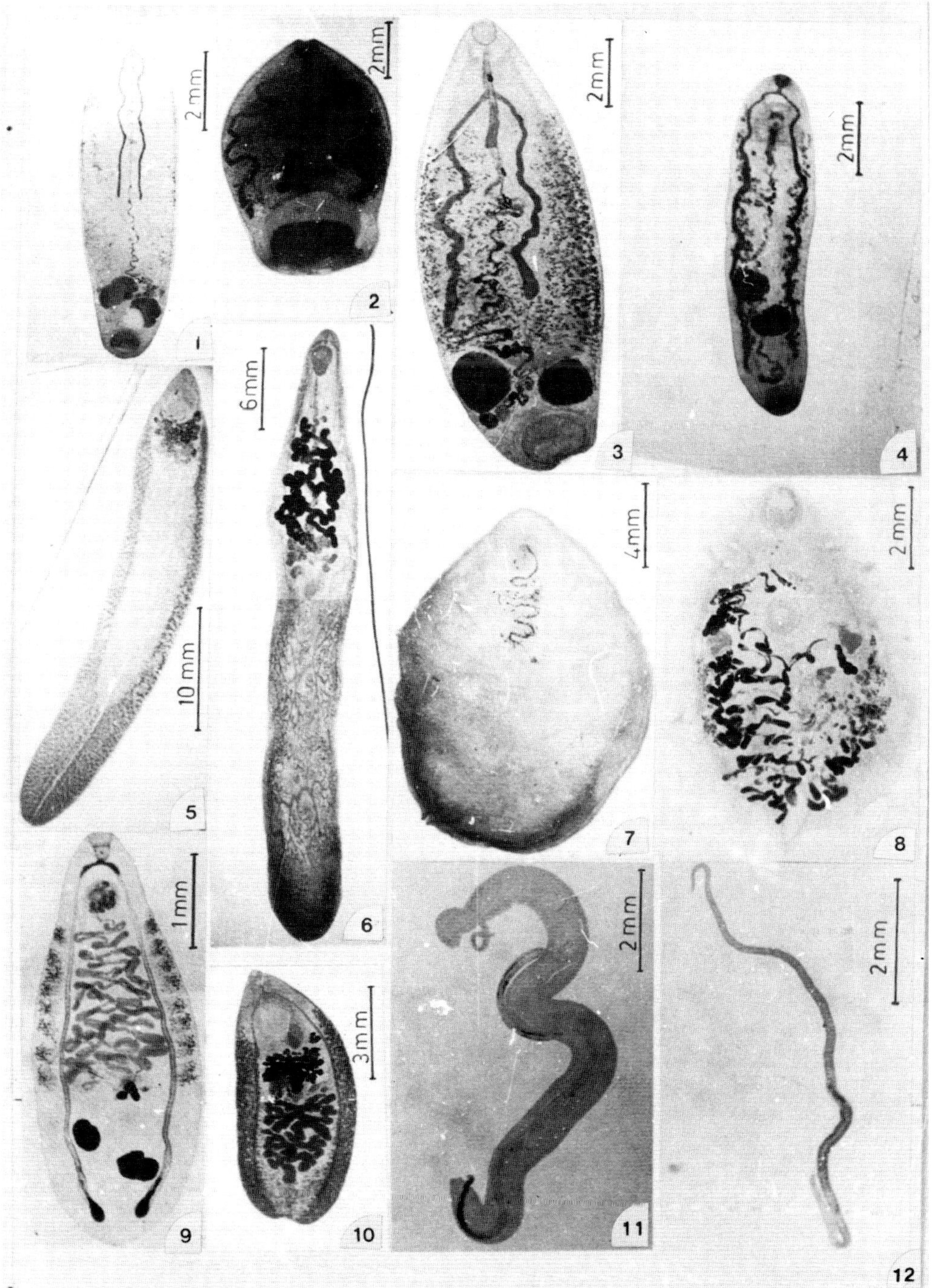

Fig. 1: *Fischoederius elongatus*; Fig. 2: *F. cobboldi*; Fig. 3: *Carmyerius spatiosus*; Fig. 4: *Velasquezotrema tripurensis*; Fig. 5: *Fasciola gigantica*; Fig. 6: *Fasciolopsis buski* (Assam origin); Fig. 7: *F. buski* (Meghalaya origin); Fig. 8: *Eurytrema pancreaticum*; Fig. 9: *Opisthorchis noverca*; Fig. 10: *Artyfechinostomum sufrartyfex*; Fig. 11: *Schistosoma indicum* (male with female); Fig. 12: *S. indicum* (female)

Classification of genera and species illustrated

Platyhelminthes: Trematoda: Digenea: Prosostomata

Family Schistosomatidae
  Subfamily Schistosomatinae
    Schistosoma indicum
Family Paramphistomidae
  Subfamily Paramphistominae
    Paramphistomum epiclitum
    P. gracile
    Calicophoron calicophorum
    C. papillosum
    C. shillongensis
    Explanatum explanatum
  Subfamily Orthocoeliinae
    Orthocoelium orthocoelium
    O. dicranocoelium
    O. scoliocoelium
    O. dawesi
    O. streptocoelium
    O. parvipapillatum
    Leiperocotyle meghalayensis
  Subfamily Cladorchiinae
    Olveria indica
    O. bosi
  Subfamily Gastrodiscinae
    Gastrodiscoides hominis
    Homalogaster paloniae
Family Gastrothylacidae
  Subfamily Gastrothylacinae
    Fischoederius elongatus
    F. cobboldi
    Gastrothylax crumenifer
    Carmyerius spatiosus
  Subfamily Velasquezotrematinae
    Velasquezotrema tripurensis
Family Fasciolidae
  Subfamily Fasciolinae
    Fasciola gigantica
  Subfamily Fasciolopsinae
    Fasciolopsis buski
Family Dicrocoeliidae
  Subfamily Eurytrematinae
    Eurytrema pancreaticum
Family Opisthorchiidae
  Subfamily Opisthorchiinae
    Opisthorchis noverca
Family Echinostomatidae
  Subfamily Echinostomatinae
    Artyfechinostomum sufrartyfex
    Echinostoma revolutum
Family Notocotylidae
  Subfamily Notocotylinae
    Catatropis indicus

References

Bali, H.S. and Fotedar, D.N. 1974. On a new amphistome, *Olveria thapari* n. sp. from the rumen of crossbred sheep from Kashmir. Indian Journal of Helminthology, 24: 30–39.

Bambroo, N. 1970. On two species of *Gastrothylax* Poirier, 1883 from sheep in Kashmir. Kashmir Science, 7: 147–155.

Dey, S., Basubaul, T., Roy, B. and Dey, D. 1989. A new rapid method using tetramethyl silane for electron microscopy: Application to the trematode parasite *Homalogaster paloniae*. Journal of Microscopy, 156: 259–261.

Dinnik, J.A. 1964. *Paramphistomum sukumum* sp. nov. and other stomach flukes from cattle in Sukumaland area of the Lake region, Tanganyika. Parasitology, 54: 201–209.

Eduardo, S.L. 1980.Taxonomic value of tegumental structure in the identification of some species of the family Paramphistomidae Fischoeder, 1901 occurring in mammals. Proc. EMOP, 3: 196.

Eduardo, S.L. 1980. *Bilatorchis papillogenitalis* n. g., n. sp. (Paramphistomidae: Orthocoeliinae), a parasite of the red lechwe (*Kobus leche* Gray, 1850) from Zambia. Systematic Parasitology, 1: 141–149.

Eduardo, S.L. 1980. *Orthocoelium indonesiense*, a new species of amphistome from ruminants in Indonesia. Systematic Parasitology, 1: 201–210.

Eduardo, S.L. 1980. A new genus, *Leiperocotyle*, for *Cotylophoron okapi* Leiper,1935 and *C. congolense* Baer, 1936 and redescription of *C. okapi*. Systematic Parasitology, 1: 255–263.

Eduardo, S.L. 1981. *Fischoederius brevisaccus*, a new species of pouched amphistome (Gastrothylacidae) from ruminants in the Philippines. *Systematic Parasitology*, 3: 1–6.

Eduardo, S.L. 1982. The taxonomy of the family Paramphistomidae Fischoeder, 1901 with special reference to the morphology of species occurring in ruminants. I. General consideration. Systematic Parasitology, 4: 7–57.

Eduardo, S.L. 1982. The taxonomy of the family Paramphistomidae Fischoeder, 1901 with special reference to the morphology of species occurring in ruminants. II. Revision of the genus *Paramphistomum* Fischoeder, 1901. Systematic Parasitology, 4: 189–238.

Eduardo, S.L. 1983. The taxonomy of the family Paramphistomidae Fischoeder, 1901 with special reference to the morphology of species occurring in ruminants. III. Revision of the genus *Calicophoron* Näsmark, 1937. Systematic Parasitology, 5: 25–79.

Eduardo, S.L. 1984. The taxonomy of the family Paramphistomidae Fischoeder, 1901 with special reference to the morphology of species occurring in ruminants. IV. Revision of the genus *Gigantocotyle* Näsmark, 1937 and elevation of the subgenus *Explanatum* Fukui, 1929 to full generic status. Systematic Parasitology, 6: 3–32.

Eduardo, S.L. 1985. The taxonomy of the family Paramphistomidae Fischoeder, 1901 with special reference to the morphology of species occurring in ruminants. V. Revision of the genus *Cotylophoron* Stiles and Goldberger, 1910. Systematic Parasitology, 7: 3–26.

Eduardo, S.L.1985. The taxonomy of the family Paramphistomidae Fischoeder, 1901 with special reference to the morphology of species occurring in ruminants. VI. Revision of the genus *Orthocoelium* (Sites & Goldberger, 1910) Price & McIntosh, 1953. Systematic Parasitology, 7: 125–158.

Eduardo, S.L. 1985. The taxonomy of the family Paramphistomidae Fischoeder, 1901 with special reference to the morphology of species occurring in ruminants. VII. Redescription of

Leiperocotyle congolense (Baer, 1936) Eduardo, 1980 and a new name, *Leiperocotyle gretillati* for *Ceylonocotyle scoliocoelium* var. *benoiti* Gretillat, 1966. Systematic Parasitology, 7: 231–238.

Jones, A. 1986. A comparative morphological study of the subfamily Gastrodiscinae Monticelli, 1892 (Paramphistomidae) with comments on some members of related subfamilies. Journal of Natural history, 20: 863–880.

Mehra, H.R. 1980. The fauna of India and adjacent countries. Manager of Publications, Govt. of India, Delhi, pp. 418.

Näsmark, K.E. 1937 Revision of the trematode family Paramphistomidae. Zoologiska Bidrag fran Uppsala, 16: 301–565.

Roy, B. and Tandon, V. 1990. On a new trematode belonging to the genus *Velasquezotrema* Eduardo, 1987 from *Bos indicus*. Zoologischer Anzeiger, 224: 106–113

Roy, B. and Tandon, V. 1990. *Leiperocotyle meghalayensis* (Paramphistomidae: Orthocoeliinae), a new species from cattle (*Bos indicus* L.) in India. Zoologischer Anzeiger, 225: 63–70.

Roy, B. and Tandon, V. 1995. *Calicophoron shillongensis* sp. n. (Trematoda, Paramphistomidae), a new parasite from the goat (*Capra hircus* L.) in India. Acta Parasitologica, 40(4); 193–197.

Sey, O. 1974. On the species of *Paramphistomum* of cattle and sheep in Hungary. Acta Veterinaria Academiae Scientiarum Hungaricae, 24: 19–37.

Sey, O. 1979. Examination of the validity and systematic position of some paramphistomids of Indian ruminants. Parasitologica Hungarica, 12: 31–36.

Sey, O. 1979. Life cycle and geographical distribution of *Paramphistomum daubneyi* Dinnik, 1962 (Trematoda: Paramphistomata). Acta Verinaria Academiae Scientiarum Hungaricae, 27: 115–130.

Sey, O. 1980. Revision of the Amphistomes of European ruminants. Parasitologica Hungarica, 13: 13–25.

Sey, O. 1980. Re–examination of an amphistome (Trematoda) collection deposited in the Geneva Museum with a description of *Orthocoelium saccocoelium* sp. n. Revue Suisse de Zoologie, 87: 431–437.

Sey, O. 1983. Revision of the family Gastrothylacidae Stiles et Goldberger, 1910 (Trematoda: Paramphistomata). Acta Zoologica Academiae Scientiarum Hungaricae, 19: 223–252.

Sey, O. 1984. Description of *Watsonius papillatus* sp. n. and the revision of the subfamily Watsoniinae Näsmark, 1937 (Trematoda: Paramphistomata). Acta Zoologica Hungarica, 30: 493–510.

Sey, O. 1984. Scanning electron microscopic examination of the tegumental surface of some amphistomes (Trematoda: Paramphistomata). Parasitologica Hungarica, 17: 45–49.

Sey, O. 1984. Amphistomes of Vietnamese vertebrates (Trematoda: Amphistomida). Parasitologica Hungarica, 17: 45–49.

Singh, K. S. 1970. On *Srivastavaia indica* n. g., n. sp. (Paramphistomidae), a parasite of ruminants and its life history. In: Singh, K.S. and Tandon, B.K. (eds.). H.D. Srivastava Commemoration volume, 117–126.

Srivastava, C.B. 1982. The fauna of India and adjacent countries. Vol. I. Manager of Publications, Govt. of India, Delhi, pp. 163.

Srivastava, H.D., Prasad, A. and Maurya, A.C. 1980. A new pouched amphistome, *Duttiella cephaloporus* gen. et sp. nov. (Family Gastrothylacidae) from buffaloes. Proceedings of National Academy of Science, India, 50(b): 4.

Verghese, C.G., Pillai, K.N., Thomas, P.C. and Peter, C.T. 1971. On the occurrence of *Haplorchis taichui* (Nishigori, 1929) Witenberg, 1930 (Trematoda: Heterophyidae) in domestic pigs (*Sus scrofa domesticus*). Japanese journal of Parasitology, 20: 406–409.

Yamaguti, S. 1971. Synopsis of digenetic trematodes of vertebrates, Vol. I & II. Keigaku Publishing Co., Tokyo, pp. 1074.

Index